Chiropractic Medicine

Chiropractic Medicine

An Ethnographic Study

Robert Hartmann McNamara

LEXINGTON BOOKS
Lanham • Boulder • New York • London

Published by Lexington Books
An imprint of The Rowman & Littlefield Publishing Group, Inc.
4501 Forbes Boulevard, Suite 200, Lanham, Maryland 20706
www.rowman.com

6 Tinworth Street, London SE11 5AL, United Kingdom

British Library Cataloguing in Publication Information Available

Library of Congress Cataloging-in-Publication Data

Names: McNamara, Robert Hartmann.
Title: Chiropractic medicine : an ethnographic study / Robert Hartman McNamara.
Description: Lanham : Lexington Books, [2019] | Includes bibliographical references and index.
Identifiers: LCCN 2018046664 (print) | LCCN 2018048340 (ebook) | ISBN 9781498591416 (Electronic) | ISBN 9781498591409 (cloth : alk. paper)
Subjects: LCSH: Chiropractic. | Alternative medicine.
Classification: LCC RZ241 (ebook) | LCC RZ241 .M36 2019 (print) | DDC 615.5/34—dc23
LC record available at https://lccn.loc.gov/2018046664

♾™ The paper used in this publication meets the minimum requirements of American National Standard for Information Sciences—Permanence of Paper for Printed Library Materials, ANSI/NISO Z39.48-1992.

Printed in the United States of America

To Dan and Mary Ann, who made all these adventures possible.

Contents

Preface

For many years I had seen a chiropractor for back problems and several providers became personal friends as a result of my role as a patient. As I continued to watch many of them struggle with the changes in health care in this country, I became interested in how chiropractors differed from physicians, particularly primary care providers. I also have friends and colleagues who are physicians and the laments offered by this group sounded similar to the complaints of chiropractors. This, coupled with my natural curiosity about exactly what chiropractors do, led me to begin exploring this topic in more depth. While I thought this topic would be a timely one, particularly given the health care reforms that are occurring in the United States, I also naively thought that chiropractors would welcome an opportunity to provide their input and opinions about the changes in medicine as they relate to their profession. What I did not realize, however, was that sociologists who had studied chiropractors in the past (albeit there were very few of them), had been highly critical of the profession and the people in it.

Thus, when I solicited the help of chiropractors to understand the issues in the profession, my requests were met with unanswered emails and phone calls from some providers, declines without explanation from others, and in the cases of my friends, some promised to participate in the study, but simply stopped taking my calls. This was very surprising and it initially made me wonder if the criticisms about chiropractors contained some element of truth: were they hiding something, were they afraid that what I would find that chiropractic treatments were a series of smoke and mirrors? While I could understand why some chiropractors did not want to participate in the study (e.g. they did not believe in research, they were unwilling to sacrifice an opportunity to earn revenue for the practice), some of these providers were friends who distanced themselves from me once they learned I was going to study the profession.

It was only after I had interviewed several chiropractors that I began to realize that many chiropractors felt defensive about outside efforts to study the profession; perhaps previous criticisms by the medical profession and/or sociologists tainted their point of view about anyone other than a chiropractor studying the population. This realization led me to organize the findings of the study from the perspective and accounts of chiropractors themselves. That is, I used the chiropractors' voices to tell the larger story and let the narrative unfold in their own words. I hope these accounts, offered by their colleagues, mentors, and friends show that my goal is to offer an objective account of the issues and is not "a hachet job" as one chiropractor offered in his assessment of this project. Rather, this study is an assessment of the issues as chiropractors themselves define and explain them.

Acknowledgments

As anyone who has conducted social science research in general, and ethnographic studies in particular understands, projects like these are rarely accomplished alone. Often the researcher(s) is indebted to colleagues, friends, family, as well as the key people involved in the population or culture under study. In my case, I am indebted to the deans and provosts who shared their extensive insight into the nature of chiropractic medicine, its history, as well as their predictions of what the future holds for the profession. I also owe all the chiropractors, physicians, physical therapists, massage therapists, insurance folks, representatives of the Joint and a host of others who graciously gave me their time so that I could gain insight into the profession and the people in it. Thank you all for what you shared with me and I hope the following pages capture the issues in a meaningful and organized way.

My colleagues, Terry Williams of the New School, along with Drs. Maria Shelley and Carrie Bucher, merit thanks for their help in organizing my thoughts and ideas about the manuscript. I would also like to thank Dr. Sean Griffin, my department head at The Citadel, for his willingness to be flexible regarding my teaching schedule during the project. Trying to interview a hundred people while managing a full-time teaching load is no small feat and Sean was very supportive over the course of the project. On the production side, Courtney Morales at Lexington Books was an enthusiastic supporter of this project and I am grateful for her encouragement and ideas.

Chapter 1

Introduction and Methods

A few months ago, I spent the weekend moving several yards of mulch around my front and back yards. By the end of the day, I was tired and sore. I woke up the next morning and realized that my back muscles were in spasm and told my wife that I was "out of alignment." As a medical professional, one who also made semi-regular use of a chiropractor, she knew that it meant I would be visiting a local chiropractor for an adjustment.

We had made use of several different chiropractors over the years to treat back and neck injuries. My first experience with a chiropractor, who was a friend at the time, involved an initial assessment, complete with x-rays and a consultation, that indicated that the curvature of my neck was insufficient and would require several treatments to restore it to normal levels. This, I was told, was causing my occasional back pain. I came back the next day and received my first adjustment.

I remember lying facedown on a table, and the chiropractor, a Logan University graduate, performed a technique called "basic" on me. This involved the chiropractor finding an area around my buttocks (I later learned there is a nerve that runs through that area), with one hand while the other pressed into the area in spasm. Then he used a series of techniques on me that resulted in loud noises from this strange table that had sections that dropped once he put pressure on that portion of my body. The spasms were alleviated, at least temporarily and some of the pain subsided. Other visits produced similar results, so I would occasionally visit this provider for treatment.

After moving to another part of South Carolina, we found another chiropractor who specialized in sports injuries. This was the provider I visited after my mulching adventure. My experiences with this chiropractor were quite different however. While there were different techniques used, there were also noticeable "audibles" from the adjustment. These cracking sounds, I later learned, were the release of gases in the body, similar to what is heard when a person cracks their knuckles. Still, it was a bit unsettling, particularly when the adjustment involved my neck. The stiffness and pain relief from these adjustments were considerable though. At times, the muscle spasm would stop almost immediately, the range of motion from the problem area would be restored, while in other cases, when the injury was severe, such as the one from my mulching experience, the problem took a day or two to resolve. I was often sore from these adjustments, and could not tell if the ice pack was to help with the initial injury, the adjustment, or both.

After being treated a few times by this chiropractor, I became curious about exactly what was going on during the treatment. These visits were very different from those involving my primary care physician, so I wondered what the chiropractor did that my regular doctor did not. During these treatments, I would allow the chiropractor to gently massage my back and then use his hands to feel along my spine area and he would invariably find a spot that triggered pain or discomfort. He would leave his finger in that spot and then use it as a marker to manipulate the area, even when I would not offer where my pain was coming from. He would also hold my feet together and bend my knees as if measuring them. That was a bit confusing too. After a few treatments, I asked, "How does this all work? How did you know where the problem was?" He would typically shrug and say "I don't know, it's all God." Wait, what?

As a Christian, I think he was trying to be humble, but I never really received a complete answer to my question. I trusted this doctor, who also became a friend, and he was making me feel better so I was willing to let it go at first, but my curiosity led me to learn more about chiropractic medicine. I have since learned that these types of comments are not uncommon from some chiropractors, in part because of the philosophy of treatment and the training they receive, and in part because there generally lacks a scientific explanation of what occurs.

As it turns out, the religious component of what this particular chiropractor said to me has been the topic of some sociological research. For instance, Meister (2010), using paradigms from the sociology of religion, offered insight into the evangelical nature of chiropractic medicine, where providers used techniques employed by high-profile pastors to convince prospective patients to visit their offices. Meister's subjects also used a form of evangelism to globally distinguish chiropractic from traditional medical treatments by physician, thereby giving it a more divine inspiration.

A third technique used by chiropractors in Meister's (2010) research involved providers using their own illnesses to serve as a kind of religious testimony, a technique also used by some evangelical pastors. These efforts were successful largely because the patients were familiar with a

Christian message and the techniques established a pastor-like trust with patients. As Meister points out, nothing in the message had anything to do with scientifically validated forms of treatment, but it did provide a platform to distinguish chiropractors from other medical doctors and, especially, from other chiropractors in the area.

The scientific validity of chiropractic treatment is controversial and there are many chiropractors who absolutely believe in the science behind the treatments, but a significant challenge for chiropractic medicine centers around the issue of whether there is adequate proof about the effectiveness of chiropractic adjustments, particularly as they compare with other forms of treatment. Some chiropractors scoff at science and other rational forms of verification in favor of the dogmatic belief that what they do, like faith, is beyond scientific inquiry. Many chiropractors from this school of thought point to the fact that patients say they feel better, thereby validating the treatment. However, patient satisfaction or the relief of symptoms is not proof that a technique worked. As critics point out, the power of suggestion and/or a placebo effect can convince a patient that they feel better. Thus, these accounts are analogous to customer satisfaction surveys, and are not an adequate substitute for scientific validity. We will return to this notion of religious faith as a part of the chiropractic experience in later chapters, where we discuss the scope of practice for chiropractors as well as the wide variability of practitioners within the profession. As we will see, such beliefs, along with an inconsistent message about what chiropractic medicine is or should be, contribute to the controversy and skepticism about the profession.

CHIROPRACTIC MEDICINE DEFINED

It may be fair to say that most people really do not understand much about chiropractic medicine or exactly what chiropractors do. If you asked an average American about chiropractic medicine, it is likely to result in an array of questions about it. In addition to the obvious questions, such as what exactly is chiropractic medicine, how does it work, and what type of people make use of this type of care, other questions about comparisons to physicians are inevitable, since that is what most people use as an identifying marker in medicine.

For those who understand a bit about traditional medicine, questions such as what types of people become chiropractors and how are they different from traditional physicians are likely, along with those that raise concerns about the level of credibility offered to chiropractors compared to physicians. Other questions could include the way chiropractors operate. These are all reasonable questions but, unfortunately, the answers to them are not nearly as straightforward or simple. As we will see, the confusing nature of chiropractic medicine can lead some people to be skeptical about treatments and providers.

In addition to these questions, there are a host of sociological questions about chiropractors and chiropractic medicine, particularly in light of the recent health care reform taking place in the United States. Other issues ripe for sociological discussion include the professional identity and social standing of chiropractors and their efforts to stake a claim as a legitimate provider of various forms of treatment. Also important for consideration are the issues and challenges involved in the training and education of chiropractors, along with the political and social issues stemming from the profession.

Similarly, the interactions and relationships between chiropractors and patients, between chiropractors and physicians, and between chiropractors and the general public also generate fascinating sociological discussions about the profession. While some of these topics have been explored by other sociologists and researchers in the past, given the numerous changes to the medical landscape in the United States, one of the goals of the present study is to understand the impact of the changes taking place in the current health care environment as they relate to chiropractic medicine.

As one advocate of chiropractic medicine involved in this study noted, there are lots of "warts," or limitations, in medicine and most providers would rather not discuss or call attention to the ones in their own field (although they may be more willing to expose them in other professions). Similarly, there are those who enter a profession with less than ethical motives and for whom economic greed drives their efforts. To suggest that all chiropractors are quacks or frauds, or to imply that what they do is either a placebo or ineffective is an unfair assessment—traditional medicine or medical doctors struggle with similar criticisms and are not without flaws. Both professions have "warts," both leave many questions unanswered about patients' health, and both continually need objective assessments of standard practices to ensure providers are offering the best care possible. The main difference between the two is that traditional medicine has continued to attempt to develop scientific explanations for the unknown aspects of medicine and until recently, chiropractic medicine has not. This has set in motion a contest of credibility for chiropractic medicine and providers within the medical community, the public, and in some cases, even each other.

What follows is a two-year exploration into the chiropractic profession, including time spent talking to chiropractors and a host of others involved in the medical field, including acupuncturists, physical therapists, primary care physicians, massage therapists, insurance company representatives, Medicare and billing specialists, orthopedic surgeons, and deans and provosts at various chiropractic colleges. The focus of this study is on South Carolina and its chiropractors, but many of the issues extend far beyond the borders of that state. While a more detailed description of the methods used for this study is offered later in this chapter, it is important to note that much of the discussions and topics outlined in this study come from practitioners themselves, with their accounts and commentary a central and driving force for much of what is coming in the chapters ahead.

WHAT IS CHIROPRACTIC MEDICINE?

Chiropractic medicine is one type of treatment that falls under the category of Complementary and Alternative Medicine (CAM). This collection of treatments, which include chiropractic medicine, acupuncture, yoga, herbal medicine, and other forms, has become increasingly popular in the United States. According to one estimate, in 1990, about a third of all Americans had used some form of CAM. By 2002, the number had nearly doubled and the numbers continue to increase even today (McMillen, 2011). Chiropractic care is perhaps the most widely known form of CAM and it too has seen increases in popularity, despite the fact that only a small segment of the population actually knows, uses, and understands it.

According to the American Chiropractic Association, the largest organization within the profession, chiropractic medicine is defined in the following way:

> Chiropractic is a health care profession that focuses on disorders of the musculoskeletal system and the nervous system, and the effects of these disorders on general health. Doctors of chiropractic—often referred to as DCs, chiropractors or chiropractic physicians—practice a drug-free, hands-on approach to health care that includes patient examination, diagnosis and treatment. In addition to their expertise in spinal manipulation/adjustment, doctors of chiropractic have broad diagnostic skills and are also trained to recommend therapeutic and rehabilitative exercises, as well as to provide nutritional, dietary and lifestyle counseling. (American Chiropractic Associaion.org, 2017)

From its very beginning, chiropractic medicine has faced challenges about the scientific validity of the treatment and the credibility of its practitioners. Since those early years, many of these criticisms have remained, but legislation, licensure, and litigation have created an environment where chiropractic care is allowed in all fifty states, and licenses are required of all chiropractors who wish to practice medicine. As the data indicates, chiropractic care, while still marginal in terms of popularity, has become more commonplace in recent years as a form of alternative treatment for people, particularly in the United States.

Evidence of the popularity of chiropractic medicine is seen in estimates that it is a $14 billion a year industry, particularly for neck and back injuries (English and Keating, 2015). Still, many critics contend that chiropractic care lacks scientific rigor, amounts to quackery and fraud, or simply is no more effective as a form of treatment than traditional remedies. While the medical community is legally prohibited from discriminating against chiropractors, there remains a significant amount of controversy and contention about chiropractic care and treatment.

THE PUBLIC'S PERCEPTION OF CHIROPRACTORS

The public seems poorly informed about what chiropractors do and the nature of chiropractic medicine. Surprisingly little data has been collected on the public's perception of chiropractors in the United States. Of what data does exist, many practitioners call attention to recent research that suggests about 14 percent of the population use a chiropractor, an increase from the 9 percent found in a 2012 study by the National Health Interview Survey.

More recently, according to a 2015 report by Gallup, entitled *Americans' Perceptions of Chiropractic*, which was a collaboration between Gallup and the Palmer College of Chiropractic, found that about 14 percent (approximately 33 million people) have visited a chiropractor in the last twelve months (English and Keating, 2015). Additionally, about half of the population had been seen by a chiropractor. Still, about as many Americans (49 percent) claim to have never seen a chiropractor. This data, in comparison to previous public opinion polls, suggests that the number of people willing to be treated by chiropractors, while still quite small, is increasing.

While this study's findings suggest more people are considering the use of a chiropractor, there are some patterns worth noting, particularly from those people who had never seen a chiropractor. For instance, among the people surveyed, younger adults (aged eighteen to thirty-four), compared to older adults (those aged thirty-five to forty-nine), are more likely to say they have never been to a chiropractor. Blacks (compared to whites or Hispanics), and men (compared to women), as well as people with higher levels of education and income (compared to those with fewer years of education or lower incomes), are more likely to have never seen a chiropractor (English and Keating, 2015).

Among those who have made use of chiropractic treatment, most people average about one visit per month. In the survey, the average number of visits within the past year was eleven. Women are slightly more likely to see their chiropractors than men (with women averaging 11.5 visits compared to men with 9.4 visits in the last year). Older people, those aged fifty to sixty-four, and those whose annual household income is between $50,000 and $100,000 report less frequent visits than users in other age and income categories (English and Keating, 2015).

In terms of why they visit a chiropractor, 60 percent of users overall said they only see a chiropractor when they are in pain (English and Keating, 2015). This is a critical issue that will be explored in greater depth in subsequent chapters since it relates to chiropractors' perceptions of their scope of practice and philosophies of treatment.

If 60 percent of users see a chiropractor only when they are in pain, this leaves about 30 percent who said they see one on a regular basis (some respondents had no opinion or were unsure how they felt about this question in the study) even if they do not have pain. This finding raises an important issue about whether the public thinks of chiropractors as primary care providers. In fact, this study found that only 10 percent of users view their chiropractor as a primary care provider, while nearly three-quarters of respondents said they did not feel this was an appropriate role for chiropractors to play.

Even nutrition and diet were topics that respondents generally did not want to talk about with their chiropractors. Thus, even among those who use chiropractors, perhaps the most informed segment of the population about chiropractic medicine and treatment, generally perceive the role of the chiropractor to only address neck and back issues and even then, only when the patient is in pain (English and Keating, 2015).

This finding is underscored by actually asking respondents how they would address neck or back pain. The question was posed to respondents that if they experienced neck or back pain, whom would they most likely see? Approximately 54 percent said they would see a medical doctor first, while about 30 percent said they would visit their chiropractor. While a small percentage of people answered that they would seek out a physical therapist or a massage therapist, these findings suggest that even chiropractic users think that chiropractors should be confined to treatment for neck and back ailments—and would still seek out their primary physician before going to a chiropractor (English and Keating, 2015).

In an attempt to gain further insight into why some adults would be reluctant to seek out chiropractic treatments, respondents were asked if they had ever been discouraged from seeking such treatment. Generally speaking, nearly two-thirds said others tried to discourage them from seeking chiropractic treatment. Clearly there remains some skepticism or concern about the danger involved in chiropractic treatment.

Perhaps this finding is due to the fact that family, friends, or physicians do not think users are making informed decisions, or perhaps they do not understand what chiropractic treatment involves. However, 70 percent of users feel they have a firm grasp of what chiropractors do. Unfortunately, these same respondents do not know the educational requirements needed to become a licensed chiropractor. Only about 15 percent of adults accurately estimated the number of years of education needed to become a chiropractor (English and Keating, 2015).

While the public generally does not really understand what chiropractors do or how someone becomes a chiropractor, this lack of understanding does not seem to affect people's overall assessment. About 50 percent of respondents agree that most chiropractors are trustworthy (39 percent state they did not know or had no opinion about the trustworthiness of members of this profession). Additionally, nearly 64 percent state they believe that most chiropractors have their patient's best interests in mind (28 percent state they did not know or had no opinion on this question). Generally speaking, these findings are consistent with previous research that those who have been treated by chiropractors are more likely to have a positive view of them (English and Keating, 2015).

Those who do not use chiropractors, however, offer a different view. About a quarter of respondents think that chiropractic care is dangerous and about a third are unsure about those risks. That uncertainty increases to 47 percent among people who have never been to a chiropractor. That is, even if people have no opinion on the danger of chiropractic treatment, if one has never been to a chiropractor, those fears are heightened.

In addition, there is also a perception that the cost of receiving treatment is too high. This may be another potential reason why so few adults seek out chiropractic care. According to this study, about 43 percent think chiropractic care is too expensive and 44 percent think it requires too many visits. Women are more likely than men to agree that chiropractic care is expensive; those with less education and those with lower incomes are more likely than those with higher education levels and incomes to think chiropractic care is expensive (English and Keating, 2015).

About half of adults who have been to a chiropractor in the last five years say they would go to the chiropractor more often if it was less expensive. These findings are in contrast with most accounts of chiropractors, who contend that their fees are far lower than office visits to physicians and their treatments are far less expensive and time consuming than traditional medicine (English and Keating, 2015).

In sum, while the general public tends to look favorably upon the chiropractic profession and its practitioners, they still remain uninformed about exactly what chiropractic medicine is and how chiropractors provide treatment. There remains a good deal of skepticism about the profession, which is undoubtedly related to this lack of understanding as well as the lack of scientific studies that prove chiropractic treatment is an effective way of addressing back and neck pain. The public tends to see chiropractors not as primary care providers, but as someone to see if they have a neck or back problem, after first going to their primary care provider. These findings are an important part of the discussion of how chiropractors see themselves, as well as their understanding of their professional identity and place in medicine.

Similar to the Gallup study, Forese and Gooding (2013) found that their sample of respondents had little understanding of the profession or the types of ailments chiropractors can treat. One of the main findings of the study was that chiropractors are relatively unrecognized by the public, either in terms of their training, the expense of chiropractic treatment, or whether the public would consider a chiropractor as an initial primary care provider.

On the positive side, respondents felt that chiropractors were generally honest and cared about their patients and most thought that chiropractic care was a relatively safe form of treatment. Where it became unclear was when respondents were asked about whether chiropractors can prescribe medication to patients, whether chiropractic care is expensive, and how the treatments offered here are different from those in physical therapy.

In short, Forese and Gooding (2013) concluded that although there were generally positive perceptions about chiropractors, as evidenced of respondents' claims that they were trustworthy and ethical in their business practices, when it came to understanding what chiropractors actually do and whether or not they would utilize a chiropractor, a large percentage had no opinion, did not know, or would only use chiropractors for specific problems, such as back or neck pain.

Unfortunately, this particular study contained several methodological flaws that raise concerns about the value of the data. While this is not to invalidate what the actual respondents said or felt, the manner in which the study was conducted raises important questions about its generalizability to anything other than those particular respondents.

THE MEDICAL COMMUNITY'S PERCEPTION OF CHIROPRACTORS

While the public may offer some confidence and trust in chiropractors and in chiropractic treatments, such confidence has not always been assigned to chiropractors or chiropractic care, in the past or in the present by the medical community (Ingraham, 2016; Long, 2013; Magner and Barrett, 1995; Singh and Ernst 2008).

For instance, critics point out that the training chiropractors receive is not on par with medical schools and the knowledge chiropractors possess to diagnose and treat illness is inadequate. Critics also point to examples of unethical marketing practices, false claims, dangerous techniques, and the exploitation of patients, who cannot adequately discern the difference between medical doctors and chiropractors or to understand the science behind chiropractic treatment. However, despite these criticisms, there is some evidence to justify chiropractic treatment as a form of treatment for some types of injuries (Paige et al., 2017).

Doctors are reluctant to refer patients to chiropractors, in part due to a lack of understanding about chiropractic medicine and in part because of the wide range of providers, some of whom engage in questionable treatments. As one doctor pointed out,

> I can't refer patients to a chiropractor because I have no idea what type of treatment they will receive. Some guys know what they are doing in terms of treating some types of neck and back injuries, but a lot of them are way out there and do goofy things that have no basis in science and don't help the patient. In fact, some of these guys could make the injury worse for that patient. I can't let my reputation be affected by that nor do I want patients getting hurt. It's not that I have anything personal against chiropractors, but the only way I am going to refer a patient to one is if I know what this guy is going to do once my patient gets to his office. And since I don't have time to investigate every chiropractor to separate the good ones from the weird ones, I simply can't take that chance.

Another doctor points out that chiropractors think all doctors are out to get them. He says,

> Listen, while there was a lawsuit many years ago because the AMA tried to shut chiropractors down, there remains this feeling that all doctors are against chiropractors or that physicians somehow feel threatened by what they do. I don't feel threatened since they are not going to take away patients from me. . . . Some of the things that I do can't be done by chiropractors and even if they could, there's no way they are going to be a threat to me—I have more work than I know how to manage as it is. But this perception that the medical community is threatened by chiropractors and so we try to cut them out of the industry is all in their heads. Maybe that's what they do to each other or that's what they might do if they were in our position, but the problem really feels to me like an example of their own inferiority complexes and they are looking for someone to blame for the fact that they haven't done what they needed to in order for society and other professions to look at them with respect.
>
> This notion that we know what chiropractors do and the only reason we don't refer to them is because we don't want to lose the fee? That's nonsense. If we can find a way to help the patient, why wouldn't we explore that? I refer patients to physical therapists all the time, technically I'm "losing" money on that unless I own that PT practice. So it's not a matter of some conspiracy or we are so economically motivated that we want to cut people out of the business. We just don't know what business they are actually in and aren't able to get good answers when we ask them.

Some chiropractors argue that the reason many doctors view chiropractors with suspicion is because of a lack of understanding of neck and back injuries. This line of thinking suggests that because non-specialist physicians do not know enough about treating such injuries, they often have poor success with patients. However, the logic behind this thinking is a bit confusing: if doctors routinely do not know how to treat neck and back injuries (unless they have specialized training such as an orthopedic surgeon), would they not make an effort to learn more about what chiropractors do? Where there may be some value to the discussion is the exposure to chiropractic treatments early in a medical student's training.

For instance, Wong's (2013) study of Canadian medical students attempted to learn more about how they perceive chiropractic treatments and other forms of CAM treatments. Wong found that about half of the students held negative attitudes about chiropractic medicine and also knew very little about it. For instance, the vast majority of medical students said they were unaware of any scientific studies of the effectiveness of chiropractic treatment and some students did not know that chiropractors engaged in treatments such as acupuncture, nutritional counseling, and other forms of treatment.

While not interested in learning chiropractic techniques, respondents in this study said they were interested in learning more about chiropractic medicine so that they could have a wider array of treatment options for their patients. This was not as much an endorsement of chiropractic by medical students as much as it was a willingness to consider a host of treatments depending on their patients' needs. From the perspective of the chiropractic community, this type of information could be used as an opportunity for physicians and chiropractors to engage in collaborative efforts and subsequently improving patients' overall health (Wong et al., 2013).

In general, the problem traditional medicine has with chiropractic care is the absence of any scientific proof that the types of treatments offered actually work. As was noted earlier, a recent article in the *Journal of the American Medical Association* (JAMA) points to the mild effectiveness of some chiropractic treatments in relieving back pain, but the problem for many physicians has been a fundamental lack of effort to validate the treatment or adequately explain the philosophy (Paige et al., 2017). As one chiropractor put it,

> One of the things I love about chiropractic is that it's been around for over a hundred years and it hasn't changed. Medicine is always changing, they weren't doing the things they do today fifty years ago and the things they'll be doing fifty years from now will be different from what they are doing today. Chiropractic principles have stood the test of time. How do I know? If it didn't work, patients wouldn't come to me over and over again.

An orthopedic surgeon who refers patients to chiropractors in his home town offers this as a testimony to the problem. He says,

> Yes, medicine has changed over time, that's because we have continued to strive for scientific answers to problems and illness. We used to put leeches on people because we thought it worked too, but we realized, after investigating further, that this actually made people worse. So our failures are not really evidence of our lack of effectiveness. Our failures are a sign that we are always trying to improve, we are always seeking the best way to treat and to scientifically determine which is the best way to get our patients healthy. Chiropractors don't do that. They fall back on anecdotal patient testimonies or dogmatic ideas that might have held sway a hundred years ago, but science and society has evolved considerably since then.
>
> If they could point to some good research that showed what they do is effective, I think more doctors would be willing to acknowledge that the profession is in need of maturation and more data, but we would at least be able to say there's something in there that shows it works. But many of these guys reject the idea of science, they reject the idea of evidence-based practices, and they reject the criticism levied against them because they don't have an answer. They keep going back to their mantra, that it works, it works, it works, despite any real proof that it does.
>
> They won't accept the idea that relieving symptoms doesn't mean the patient is cured, that they say they feel better is not proof that the treatment worked . . . AT ALL. And this is where they get into trouble and lose many doctors' confidence in what it is they do. So I would say that most doctors, and I'm in the small minority of people who do refer some patients to chiropractors, but most doctors either think of chiropractors as quacks, as frauds, or as so blindly misguided in their thinking that they can't be trusted, and surely not with one of our patients.

TRADITIONAL MEDICINE AND CHIROPRACTIC CARE

In addition to the skepticism from physicians about chiropractic medicine, including from groups like the American Medical Association (AMA), health care reform presents a host of challenges to the profession. Similar to medical doctors who own and operate small general medical practices, who are forced to merge with other providers to extract reasonable reimbursement rates from insurance companies, many chiropractic offices, who overwhelmingly remain solo practitioners or consist of practices with less than three providers, struggle to keep up with the outcome and accountability measures as part of the insurance reimbursement protocols. The difference, however, is that unlike the groups created to advocate for doctors or dentists, chiropractors remain decentralized and unable to marshal significant political leverage to address the changing legislative, health care, and insurance landscapes.

The implementation of the Affordable Care Act, also known as Obamacare, has changed the way insurance companies provide reimbursement for services by medical providers. With a greater emphasis on administratively documenting how and in what ways a particular form of treatment actually improves a patient's health, coupled with a greater level of restriction on the types of services medical providers can offer without justification and authorization, many medical providers have had to reexamine the services they provide, and how they operate (AMGA, 2016). For chiropractors in particular, who tend to treat patients with a more holistic approach to improve patient health, coupled with the lingering conflicts with traditional medicine (making it unlikely chiropractors will be included in collaborations with other medical providers), restrictions on the number and types of treatment they can provide have created difficulties within some practices.

SOCIOLOGY AND CHIROPRACTIC MEDICINE

A review of the literature shows a handful of studies about the sociological dimensions of the chiropractic profession or its providers (Wardell, 1952, 1955, 1961, 1968, 1976, 1978; McCorkle, 1961; Roebuck and Hunter, 1972; Lin, 1972; Rosenthal, 1986; Villenueva-Russell, 2005, 2008, 2009; Briggs, 1997; Yesalis et al., 1980; Wild, 1978; Kelmer, Hall, and Coulter, 1980), most of which occurred in the 1970s and 1980s. However, very little research has been done since 2000 and none have been conducted about how the changes in medicine, particularly as it relates to health care reform, impact chiropractors and their practices.

This lack of sociological research is a bit odd, given the many issues and challenges in health care as well as a growing body of literature on alternative medicine. Even the unethical practices of some medical providers, which would likely attract criminologists and those who study deviant behavior, would likely generate some sociological attention, not to mention medical sociology as a subfield is the largest one in the discipline. However, this has not been the case. In fact, a review of medical sociology textbooks shows scant attention devoted to chiropractors and chiropractic medicine, often just a few paragraphs (see, for instance, Cockerham, 2017). Far more attention is paid in these textbooks to faith healers and more obscure practitioners.

The earliest sociological studies on chiropractic medicine were those by Wardell (1950). In his book *The Sociology of Chiropractic*, Rosenthal (1986) pointed out that up until 1950, there were only seven sociological studies on chiropractic medicine. Much of what had been understood about the profession during a period that spanned almost twenty years was based only on Wardell's work.

These initial sociological explorations of chiropractic medicine were linked to the study of deviant behavior and this was the framework in which sociology began to examine chiropractic medicine. In the 1950s Walter Wardell offered insight into chiropractic medicine in terms of its marginality. As he described it, marginality as a concept carries with it challenges to legitimacy and credibility, along with questions about competence and inferiority. This marginality comes, according to Wardell, as a result of comparisons to traditional medicine. At the microlevel, Wardell (1952) found a good deal of role ambiguity among chiropractors and role strain in their actual performance.

Research in the 1960s and 1970s

Dimensions of the marginality of chiropractic medicine was found in work by McCorkle (1961) as well as by Roebuck and Hunter (1972) who provided insight into the dubious and outright fraudulent practices by chiropractors. Interestingly, the total number of studies published between 1950 and 1972 consisted of seven articles, four of which were authored by Wardell (Wardell, 1952; 1955; 1961; 1968). Sternberg's (1961) doctoral dissertation was a sociological study of chiropractic students and it too focused on the marginality of the profession. Lin's (1972) dissertation was the first to really question the stigma and deviant label attributed to chiropractors and he wondered if this was ever a fair appraisal of the profession.

Rosenthal (1986) attributes the early conceptualization of chiropractic as deviant behavior based on the relationship between sociology and traditional medicine. Given the political and social climate of traditional medicine, particularly its opposition to chiropractic treatment, a perception was created that chiropractic medicine was substandard and inferior to what physicians offered patients.

Research in the 1970s and 1980s

Throughout the 1970s and into the 1980s, the research began to focus less on chiropractic medicine's place in the occupational scheme and more on what chiropractors actually did and how they did it (Rosenthal, 1986; Wild, 1978; Yesalis et al., 1980; Coulter et al., 1980). For instance, in an ethnographic study of chiropractic medicine, Cowie and Roebuck (1975) offer insight into the nature of social interaction within a chiropractic office. Serving as a member of the staff, Cowie was able to observe how and in what ways the front office learned about the patients' needs, interests, and issues, and then relayed them to the doctor prior to receiving their treatment.

Drawing heavily on a Goffmanian framework, particularly as it relates to the notion of impression management and controlling the patient's understanding of the role of the chiropractor, this study offered great insight into how marketing efforts are employed, where staff members routinely encouraged patients to refer their friends and relatives to the office for care. While this may also occur in a traditional physician's office, Cowie and Roebuck point out that there is an intentionality and intensity to this type of self-promotion that can create an uncomfortable atmosphere and cause patients to question the motives of a chiropractor.

At the same time, chiropractors also attempt to provide a distinction in the type of care they provide compared to physicians. By providing a safe and sympathetic atmosphere, one that is often at odds with the patient experience in traditional doctor's offices, Cowie and Roebuck (1975) conclude that there is an element of trust that is created between the patient and the provider, including the office in general, that allows them to thoughtfully consider the advice offered by the chiropractor during their visits. In addition, like the earlier studies, much of the impression management performed by the chiropractor is an effort to manage the stigma of being a member of a "tainted" profession.

As Rosenthal (1986) points out, a second view of chiropractic medicine, which began in the late 1970s, centered on chiropractic's tension with the American Medical Association in general and physicians in particular, a tension that still exists to some extent today. Rosenthal (1986) takes a slightly different approach to this perspective by applying a framework borrowed from organizational deviance to chiropractic medicine based on his study of chiropractors in Nebraska.

In the 1980s, there was also an increased interest in sociological inquiry of chiropractic medicine, particularly outside of the United States. In Canada, Kelmer, Hall, and Coulter (1980) took issue with Wardell's position on chiropractic medicine and attempted to clarify some of the inaccuracies about chiropractic medicine. In contrast to much of the sociological literature on chiropractic medicine, which is admittedly sparse, Coulter's (1983) work is particularly noteworthy as he raises questions about the sociological understanding of chiropractic medicine and the profession.

For instance, Coulter (1983) is consistently critical of Wardell's work that characterizes the chiropractic profession as marginalized or deviant. Coulter also argues that this conceptualization, which is based more on comparing chiropractic medicine to traditional medicine than any actual data indicating marginalization, had a resonating effect on subsequent sociological studies of chiropractors and the profession. In fact, Coulter (1991) argues that such a portrayal could have shaped the general public's understanding of the profession.

Such a perspective, which calls attention to the ability of researchers to discover notions of objective truth, Coulter deserves credit for calling attention to the "taken for granted" approach the discipline has used with regard to the study of chiropractic medicine. Coulter also deserves credit for one of the earliest assessments of the role of chiropractic medicine within a changing health care landscape (2004).

Other research in the 1980s focused on how chiropractic medicine fit within the larger health care delivery of services. Rosenbaum (1986), for instance, outlined some of the factors that separate medicine from chiropractic in terms of the two professions' efforts at image enhancement.

During this period, several books were published on the chiropractic industry, but none had a specific sociological focus. Much of the work during this time continued to focus on it as a form of deviant behavior. Drawing heavily on some of the more dubious practices by chiropractors, many observers looked upon the profession in a manner similar to con artists and those who attempted to defraud the public.

Research in the 1990s and 2000s

Since the 1980s, much of the sociological research on chiropractic medicine has focused on the profession's ability to adapt and respond to the criticisms of the effectiveness of chiropractic treatments. Much of the medical literature during this period focused on evidence-based practices, meaning treatments are given much greater credibility and support when there is clinical research that shows its overall effectiveness. Clearly, this is problematic for chiropractic treatments since the lack of scientific evidence supporting these treatments has been a consistent criticism. This is particularly true of the identification and proof of the vertebral subluxation, a key element to the justification of chiropractic medicine from its very beginnings.

Like Wardell's work in the 1950s, one or two sociologists dominated the chiropractic discussions since the 1980s. However, unlike the criticisms offered by Wardell, these researchers attempted to identify key issues within the profession, particularly as they relate to health care as well as challenges within the profession. For instance, Villenueva-Russell (2005) offered insight into how chiropractic medicine has responded to the growing trend toward evidence-based practices as an assessment protocol.

As guidelines were being developed for evidence-based medicine, all complementary and alternative-based medicines, but particularly chiropractic, with its emphasis on concepts such as "vitalism" and "innate intelligence" struggled to find a place in the discussion. Consequently, chiropractic medicine's credibility and professionalism within medicine continued to suffer. The lack of evidence about chiropractic treatment also created challenges within the profession as it related to insurance reimbursement under the managed care model. This lack of understanding or willingness to embrace a scientific approach is not simply a criticism from outside the profession.

Recent research supports the idea that many chiropractors, even those who are in training at chiropractic colleges, are not as familiar with evidence-based treatment as they would like. A 2015 study of nearly 1,500 chiropractors, two-thirds of whom had been in practice for more than ten years, found that while providers had favorable attitudes toward an evidence-based approach, far less actually practiced it, citing a lack of time to develop an understanding of how to use it (Schneider et al., 2015).

Briggs (1997), a sociologist at the University of Saskatchewan, studied the philosophy of chiropractors in Canada. Despite the fact that most were trained at a single chiropractic college, the Canadian Memorial Chiropractic College in Toronto, Briggs found significant differences in chiropractors' philosophies and scope of practice. She found, for example, that about 18 percent of respondents rejected the traditional chiropractic philosophy espoused by D. D. and B. J. Palmer, and placed greater value of the scientific validation of chiropractic concepts within a narrow scope, such as musculoskeletal problems of the neck and back.

About a quarter of chiropractors surveyed adopted the traditional chiropractic philosophies and held a narrow view of a chiropractor's scope of practice. Briggs also found significant differences in chiropractic philosophy and scope of practice by province, with Quebec chiropractors more likely to espouse liberal views while Saskatchewan chiropractors hold more conservative approaches to chiropractic medicine. These are significant findings since it inhibited the ability of the country and the profession to develop effective and consistent guidelines for the treatment of patients. While this topic will be discussed at length in a subsequent chapter, much of Briggs's work focuses on developing a more sociological understanding of the profession (Briggs, Hay, and Mierau, 1997).

Despite recent efforts to enhance the credibility of the profession, significant challenges remain. For instance, Villenueva-Russell (2009) discusses a number of fundamental and historical challenges within chiropractic medicine, where there exists a school of thought that takes a more profit-centered approach to the profession than establishing its scientific credibility. While not deviant, per se, such a position does little to enhance the credibility of the profession as a patient-centered, health care provider.

As she points out, this entrepreneurial perspective was the central focus in the development of chiropractic medicine and impacted the public's trust by not following the more conventional processes used by traditional medicine to garner credibility and legitimacy. While some might consider this unconventional approach to be consistent with its founding ideology, especially in its early years, chiropractic distanced itself from interest in issues such as licensure as a mark of professionalism in favor of support from its patients. In what could be argued as a misguided attempt to redefine professionalism and its benchmarks, chiropractic medicine may have hampered its ability to achieve its original goals, namely to be considered equal to traditional medicine and physicians (Villenueva-Russell, 2008).

There appears to be some evidence in the literature and in the practices of chiropractic colleges around the country that the profession may be willing to accept the idea that in order to gain any level of credibility, like osteopaths of a generation before them, they must recognize that the philosophies of the past cannot be proven in a valid, objective, and scientific way. To that end, some chiropractic colleges began collecting data on effective treatments of back and neck injuries.

In addition to the issue of shifting its focus away from profits as a goal, chiropractors continue to wrestle with questions of credibility in the minds of the general public. For example, Villenueva-Russell (2009) offers insight into the continued understanding of chiropractic as a marginalized profession in her work on the public's perception of chiropractic medicine based on media reports. Calling attention to the notion of moral panics and the subsequent fear that such a movement generates, she points out that the highlighted cases of injuries to patients by chiropractors, particularly strokes suffered as a result of cervical manipulation (adjustments to the neck), only serve to perpetuate the perception of chiropractic as a questionable science.

This negative perception is reinforced by the profession's lack of organized response in refuting these claims and creates a type of fear that impedes chiropractic medicine's ability to be seen as legitimate. That many more patients die at the hands of medical doctors each year is overlooked or managed more effectively by the medical profession should not be lost on chiropractors. However, the public's understanding of the profession and of its treatments is skewed by its lack of access to more detailed information (Villeneuva-Russell, 2009).

Since the 1990s, there remains a lingering influence of chiropractic as a form of deviance, largely due to the questionable practices of some providers, who push the boundaries of a reasonable standard of effective care, and in part because of the inability of the profession to organize itself in a meaningful and consistent way. Villenueva-Russell (2011) offers insight into the cultural and social issues within the profession, particularly as efforts by chiropractic colleges and the profession attempt to integrate themselves with traditional medicine. Such an approach clashes with practitioners, who are often opposed to such changes, believing it would cause chiropractic medicine to be absorbed by traditional medicine and lose its distinctiveness and viability.

Further complicating the debate between the practical side of chiropractic and its academic side is the issue of which organizations, if any, have the authority to dictate the boundaries of what is considered acceptable practice.

We will return to this topic in a subsequent chapter, as it remains a central issue in understanding the social and cultural identity of the chiropractic profession.

Other studies focus on the self-perception of chiropractors in their ability to treat patients. Joan et al.'s (2004) study of experienced chiropractors in Texas offers insight into how chiropractors see their abilities to treat an assortment of illnesses and injuries, particularly unconventional illnesses, such as asthma, pregnancy, and liver and kidney ailments. Part of the success, as these respondents see it, is based on the close relationship and trust that is developed between patient and provider, something that participants believe happens less frequently with traditional medicine (Joan et al., 2004).

It was also during this period, the 1990s and into the early 2000s, that many books were written heavily criticizing the profession, particularly those written by chiropractors themselves. While not sociological in scope, and while these authors did not provide sufficient data to document their criticisms against the profession, there were sociological elements and concepts to consider in these texts. For example, in the book entitled *Spin Doctors*, Benedetti and MacPhail (2002), two investigative journalists, offer a scathing overview of the chiropractic profession and its lack of scientific validation. They also dedicate a significant amount of attention to chronicling the fraudulent, questionable, and even dangerous practices performed by chiropractors. Similarly, other accounts offered by chiropractors and scientists provide a platform of criticism of the profession and the lack of proof about chiropractic medicine as a legitimate form of treatment (Long, 2013; Magner and Barrett, 1995; Singh and Ernst, 2008).

With the exception of Villenueva-Russell's (2005; 2008; 2011) work, sociological studies since the late 1990s are largely absent in the literature. In fact, much of the research on chiropractic medicine now focuses on the clinical trials (or those studies that lack sufficient methodological rigor) on the effectiveness of spinal manipulation treatment (SMT) compared to other forms of treatment, including doing nothing at all.

The current study, then, takes some of the issues discussed in previous sociological studies and examines them in light of the health care reform that is currently being debated in the United States. The fact that some of the issues continue to plague the profession is important, as are the new issues that are topics of discussion among American chiropractors. Included in this study is a focus on the internal strife within the profession, the impact of a large-scale social problem, health care reform, as well as how and in what way chiropractic colleges are responding to changes in medicine. Included in this discussion is the shift in focus by some chiropractic colleges to train students to become primary care providers instead of traditional chiropractors. This is a very controversial issue within the profession as are the escalating costs of student debt to receive training as a chiropractor, which may explain some of the consistent declines in enrollments at most chiropractic colleges around the country.

THE PROJECT

This study attempts to explore the life of chiropractors in light of all the historical and current changes taking place within the medical profession. It also seeks to understand the external and internal threats posed to chiropractors, with an eye toward understanding how and in what ways the future of medicine, as well as their visions for the profession in the future, will alter what we currently understand to be chiropractic care. Some providers have noted that the profession will have to become better organized to establish an identity; find a way to mainstream with traditional medicine (as more chiropractic colleges appear to be doing); relegate themselves to technicians who perform a limited array of treatments for back and neck pain, but do not really serve as primary health care providers; or disband all together.

A host of issues are generated from any one of these possible scenarios and there appears to be less optimism within the profession about its future. This is particularly true since many other health care providers, such as physical therapists, osteopathic doctors, and even some types of massage therapists, can often provide a similar type of treatment offered by chiropractors. Despite the concerns and challenges within the profession, according to the U.S. Department of Labor, the chiropractic profession is growing at a much faster than average trajectory than other professions (U.S. Department of Labor Statistics, 2015). Despite this optimism, given the costs involved in completing chiropractic training (which can cost between $150,000 and $200,000, as much as medical school) coupled with the low salary (recent data from the U.S. Department of Labor Statistics shows that the median salary for a chiropractor is $64,440 per year and other data indicates that it could be lower), along with the challenges of starting and sustaining an individual practice (with considerable start-up costs along with the challenges of generating a large patient base when most chiropractors are operating as solo practitioners), these obstacles are formidable ones.

This is particularly true in light of the recent development of large chiropractic chains such as the Joint, that offer spinal and neck adjustments at a fraction of the cost of a traditional provider. In light of all these challenges, how are chiropractors coping? What are some of the real and potential consequences of these changes and how are existing providers, even successful ones, managing these turbulent times? As Medicare requirements increase the amount of documentation and verification that certain treatments are medically necessary and add to the workload of providers, not to mention the decline in reimbursement rates, it is possible that many chiropractors decide to close their practices. It is also possible that the difficulties of sustaining a practice, along with the competition for patients among providers, cause some chiropractors to engage in questionable practices and treatments in order to diversify and generate revenue. The Office of Inspector General's 2016 report about Medicare fraud pays a great deal of attention to some of these practices by chiropractors.

An Ethnographic Approach

This ethnographic study used classic techniques of systematic observation and unstructured and semi-structured interviews patients (Lecomte and Schensul, 2012; Taylor, 2002) of South Carolina chiropractors, their staff, and, to learn more about the nature of chiropractic care and how the proposed changes in health care impact the profession's viability. Time was spent in numerous chiropractic offices learning about the procedures used in operating a practice, observing interactions between staff and patients, as well as the role of the chiropractor within the practice. Formal interviews were conducted with staff members, patients, and providers, along with informal conversations that occurred as a normal part of the ethnographic approach. Visits to various chiropractic offices occurred twice a week for approximately eighteen months, with each visit lasting approximately three to four hours, including the interviews.

Some practices, for example, focus on certain segments of the patient population, such as pregnant women, sports injuries, pediatrics, or family practices, which involve an entire family seeing the provider for wellness care. Other differences focus on how potential patients are identified, through referrals, social media, online marketing, or practice-building seminars designed to enhance revenue and the size of the practice. On several occasions, while making observations in waiting rooms, informal conversations with patients occurred, to gage their understanding of chiropractic medicine, the services offered by the provider, and their overall feelings about the benefits of treatment.

Additionally, phone interviews were conducted with provosts, deans, and faculty at several schools of chiropractic medicine to learn more about the training that students receive. Given that the philosophies of a particular chiropractic college drive the nature of the medical practices of its graduates, it is also important to understand how the various chiropractic colleges and their faculty and staff socialize students to understand what chiropractic care looks like along with their professional futures in the changing face of medicine in this country.

Interviews were also conducted with members of other related professions, such as physical therapists, osteopathic doctors, and acupuncturists, to learn more about how they understand the role of chiropractors in relation to what they do compared to their own profession. Interviews were also conducted with medical doctors, including specialists such as orthopedic surgeons, general practitioners/family practice doctors, and others in the profession who could be likely to refer patients to chiropractors based on the nature of the injury or illness. Their perspective was designed to gain some insight into the nature of how the medical community generally perceives chiropractors and the range of treatments, if any, that they feel chiropractors have to offer.

Additionally, because chiropractic care must still contend for legitimacy in medicine, in order to understand the real and potential political frames that exist around medical care in general and chiropractic care in particular, attempts were made to interview advocates and critics of chiropractic treatment, including members from the American Chiropractic Association, the International Chiropractic Association and the National Association of Chiropractors, and the Federation of World Chiropractors. Their observations and commentary would have provided a greater level of insight into the political dimensions of the profession. In fact, at the 2017 conference in Washington, DC, the American Chiropractic Association made an attempt to consolidate the wide disparity within the profession with a statement about the scope of practice for its members. This was a landmark moment for the profession because until recently, the organization and others like it were reluctant to take a stand on the issue related to some type of boundary to which all chiropractors must adhere.

Finally, in an effort to understand more about the questionable practices of some chiropractors, interviews were conducted with representatives from Medicare concerning the auditing process and efforts to bring some level of accountability to the billing for chiropractic care. This was an important part of the discussion with providers since the penalties derived from audits mean that chiropractors could have to pay back some of the fees for which they were reimbursed. An understanding of the process and the extent of the problem was critical to the project since it has become a central feature of life for most chiropractors.

In sum, face-to-face and telephone interviews were conducted for this project, each lasting approximately one to two hours, and covered a range of activities and issues that span the discussion of chiropractic medicine. Additionally, numerous informal conversations occurred with practitioners and others associated with the medicine occurred over the course of the project. In total, approximately one hundred interviews and conversations occurred from Fall 2016 through Fall 2017. In the interest of maintaining confidentiality and anonymity, all identifiers of participants were removed. In their place, pseudonyms were used.

Additionally, statistical information was collected on the number of chiropractors who renewed their licenses in South Carolina during Fall 2016 and Fall 2017. This information was obtained from the Department of Labor, Licensing and Regulation, which provides administrative oversight of the licensure of chiropractors in the state. Interviews with administrative staff from this agency were also collected, who offered insight into the possible reasons for the significant decline in providers.

The formal interviews were taped, transcribed, and analyzed using The Ethnograph, a statistical software package that allows researchers to search and identify patterns and trends in texts and other documents. Notes were taken during the informal conversations with staff, providers, and patients, along with others in related fields. These notes were also entered into the software package, detailing issues, problems, trends, and other issues relating to the profession.

Challenges to the Project

Obviously there is an element of self-selection involved in this study since regular patients are only returning because they feel what they receive is beneficial, but to be fair, there is an element of self-selection in any field research project. In this case, only those providers willing to discuss the project returned phone calls and scheduled time for interviews and observations. There are segments of the chiropractic community who do not feel empirical validation is important, are overly concerned with offering insight about the nature of the profession, or simply were not interested in participating in the study. Perhaps this was due to a heavy patient load, but given that most chiropractors do not see patients every day, if they were interested in the project or in offering their insight, they could have easily made time for it. Like the self-selection issue with providers, only those deans and provosts who were interested in the larger issues returned phone calls and participated in the interviews. Some colleges have reputations for being less evidence based and less interested in understanding why chiropractic care works and thus may not have been interested in discussing the issues.

None of the participants received any compensation for participating in the study and the nature of the questions essentially focused on their opinions about the profession as well as how they structured and operated their practices. Most of the time there was some initial concern about how the information was going to be used, likely a result of some fear about the profession being disparaged in some way, but after the initial meeting, most of those concerns were dissipated. Additionally, all identifiers are changed in the context of their comments. In those instances, where it could be possible to identify a particular person, such as a dean of a particular chiropractic college, efforts were made to conceal the name and description of the institution as well as the identity of the particular person. The same is true with identifying a particular practice—in those instances where the location or the person might be recognized, descriptions are sufficiently generic to avoid the possibility of revealing the nature of the practice or the people in it.

In every case, the author is the only person who knew the identities and locations of participating practices. All the interviews were transcribed and the data was analyzed only by the author, then erased, thus ensuring anonymity and confidentiality throughout the project. This compartmentalization was important for many reasons as, we will discuss, chiropractors can be a bit concerned about their privacy and issues relating to maligning their profession. While I did my best to capture their points of view and understand the issues in an objective way, any inaccuracies, errors, important omissions, or other weaknesses of the study are mine alone.

Like many ethnographic studies, this was a labor-intensive project. Beginning in Fall 2016 and lasting throughout Fall 2017, interviews and observations were made across the state of South Carolina. The project began with obtaining a list of local chiropractors, drafting a letter of introduction and following up with a phone call to determine if the provider was interested in participating in the study. Because so many chiropractors are at the mercy of their schedules, this proved to be a time-intensive process. It was not uncommon to make eight to ten follow-up phone calls to offices and to supplement them with emails that contained a brief abstract of the project, before being able to actually talk to a chiropractor. Even then, there needed to be some context provided during that initial phone call since many did not read the abstract or were not familiar with empirical research or field research in particular.

There were also numerous cancellations and rescheduling of visits for a variety of reasons and there were routine cancellations of the interviews because a patient showed up in need of care. While some observations of patients were made as part of their normal visit, none of the conversation focused on their names or their patient histories. Most of the time the chiropractor limited the discussion to the particular patient complaint or describing the different ways to prevent illnesses or injuries as part of a standard script offered to all patients.

In Chapter 2, we look at the history of chiropractic medicine. While a fascinating topic by itself, the discovery of chiropractic treatment is intermingled with religion, science, and efforts to understand how the human body functions. The discovery of the vertebral subluxation, or dislocation of spinal vertebrae, is a central feature of the history of chiropractic medicine and remains an important element within the profession today. In fact, it may be that the history of the profession and the efforts to fend off legal challenges have evolved into what some in the profession call *philosophical issues*, or the dogma that hampers chiropractors from the credibility they seek with others in the medical profession.

In Chapter 3, we offer insight into the key participants in the study and how chiropractors practice chiropractic medicine. While there are a host of different ways to operate a practice, based in part on one's training, philosophy, perceived scope of practice, ethics, and other factors, there is a general rhythm to a chiropractic office, both from the patient's perspective and from the operational side of the provider.

To the casual observer, many elements of a practice provide key insight into the provider's philosophy of treatment and how he/she approaches patients. Most chiropractors care about their patients' health and improving their quality of life. Thus, the notion that chiropractors are calculating and motivated only by profit, while likely true in some cases, in as much as this could be argued in every profession, was not a consistent theme observed during the study.

Rather, the providers usually knew a lot about their patients, were engaging, educationally oriented, and encouraging. Within this chapter is also a discussion of the autonomy issues relating to the type of people that become chiropractors. As the title of this book suggests, chiropractors tend to be independent-minded, who prefer to act alone and have complete control over how they treat patients and how they organize their practices.

While this could be said of all physicians or small business owners, chiropractors are indeed similar to Mustang horses, who tend not to embrace the constraints of normal professions. As we learn more about chiropractors and how they approach their profession, this notion of independence and autonomy become salient features in the discussions, particularly as it relates to the challenges of identity and credibility within the profession.

In Chapter 4 we extend that description of chiropractors and include a discussion of topics such as scope of practice and philosophy of treatment, along with issues of identity within the profession. It is here that we begin to see some of the internal challenges that hamper the profession from a unifying collective voice and an inability to raise awareness about the value and legitimacy of the profession to the general public, policymakers, and medicine in general.

Issues including a lack of professional identity, internal strife within the profession, concerns about providers who mislead patients, the mistrust of other providers, who are competitors and who have been known to steal patients, staff members, and engagement in unscrupulous practices, will also be explored. It is also here that the issue of autonomy becomes so central to the reason why chiropractors remain solo practitioners instead of merging with other providers to enhance the reimbursement rates. Also within this discussion will be an assessment of the many political organizations that have been created to address the wide range of philosophies within the profession.

In Chapter 5, another issue within the profession is identified: The Joint. This large-scale effort to introduce affordable care to patients without the use of insurance and in the absence of traditional diagnostic procedures such as the x-ray and extensive patient history is a revolutionary model with the chiropractic profession. Largely controversial, many chiropractors feel as though the Joint has become the "Walmart" or "McDonald's" of chiropractic medicine and its place, while inevitable, continues to hamper efforts at achieving credibility. Advocates of the Joint, however, feel that their efforts not only elevate the profile of chiropractic to audiences that might never seek chiropractic care, but also provide an affordable way of maintaining their overall health through the many benefits of chiropractic treatment.

In Chapter 6, we focus on the training that chiropractors receive and how chiropractic colleges contribute to the scope of practice and the role that chiropractors could play within medicine. It is here that we begin to see glimpses of the variability within the profession, graduates' expectations for their careers, and the issues in higher education that impact the profession. It is also in this context that we see efforts to splinter the profession into what have been identified as three specific camps: Straights, Mixers, and Reformists. The latter is considered an integrative approach, where chiropractors are trained like doctors, while the former two are essentially philosophical camps, which retain its history and commitment to the core principles upon which the profession was founded.

In Chapter 7, the focus shifts to larger issues within the profession, such as health care reform and the many changes that are taking place in medicine in the United States. It is here that we also discuss the problems chiropractors have with insurance companies, reimbursement issues, Medicare audits, and the notion of the cash pay system.

Finally, Chapter 8 offers some theoretical insight into the nature of this profession and the challenges it faces. The work of Emile Durkheim, whose notion of trust and solidarity provides a glimpse of what might happen if the profession were to resolve its internal issues and provide some significant mechanism for social cohesion, along with enhancing the public's understanding of the role and value of chiropractors, is discussed.

REFERENCES

American Chiropractic Association, 2017. *Patient Fact Sheet.* Available at https://www.acatoday.org/Portals/60/Docs/Patients/Patient%20Fact%20Sheets/HealthyLiving_GetHealthywithChiro.pdf

AMGA, 2016. Affordable Care Act Implementation and Information. Available at https://amga.org/wcm/advocacy/issues/aca_issues.aspx

Briggs, L., Hay, D. and Mierau, D. 1997. "Canadian chiropractors' attitudes towards chiropractic philosophy and scope of practice: Implications for the implementation of clinical practice guidelines." *Journal of Canadian Chiropractic Association* 41(3): 145–154. Available at https://www.ncbi.nlm.nih.gov/pmc/articles/PMC2485157/pdf/jcca00027-0019.pdf

"Chiropractic Personnel in the 21st Century Depends on Strategy Today." 2000, *Topics in Clinical Chiropractic* 7(1): 11.

Cowie, J. B. and J. Roebuck. *An Ethnographic Study of a Chiropractic Clinic.* New York: The Free Press.

English, C. and Keating, E. 2015. "Majority in U.S. say Chiropractic Works for Neck, Back Pain." *Gallup.* Available at http://www.gallup.com/poll/184910/majority-say-chiropractic-works-neck-back-pain.aspx

Firman, G. and M. Goldstein. 1975. "The Future of Chiropractic: A Psychological View." *New England Journal of Medicine* 293: 639–642.

Forese, J. and Gooding, T. 2013. "Opinions of Chiropractors and the Chiropractic Profession from the Perspective of the Public at Large: An Exploratory Survey." *Journal of Philosophy, Principles, and Practice of Chiropractic,* December 16.

Gold, M. 1977. "A Crisis of Identity: The Case of Medical Sociology." *Journal of Health and Social Behavior* 18: 160–168

Ingraham, P. 2016. "Does Chiropractic Work?" *Pain Science.* Available at http://www.painscience.com/articles/does-chiropractic-work.php.

Joan, K. L., Richard, H. P., Rupert, R., and Daniel, D. 2004. "A living history—A qualitative study of experienced chiropractors treating visceral conditions." *Forum: Qualitative Social Research* 5: 3.

Kelner, M., Hall, O. and I. Coulter. 1980. *Chiropractors: Do They Help?* Toronto: Fitzhenry and Whiteside.

Langlois, J. K., Parrish, R. H., Rupert, R. and Dwain, D. 2004. "A Living History: A Qualitative Study of Experienced Chiropractors Treating Visceral Conditions." *Forum Qualitative Social Research* 5(3): Art 17. Available at http://www.qualitative-research.net/fqs

Lin, P. 1972. *The Chiropractor, Chiropractic and Process: A Study of the Sociology of an Occupation.* Unpublished Ph.D. Dissertation, University of Missouri.

Lisi, A. J. and Brandt, C. A. 2016. "Trends in the Use and Characteristics of Chiropractic Services in the Department of Veterans Affairs." *Journal of Manipulative Physiological Therapies* 39: 381–386.

Long, P. H. 2013. *Chiropractic Abuse: An Insider's Lament.* New York: American Council on Science and Health.

Magner, G. and Barrett, S. 1995. *Chiropractic: The Victim's Perspective*. New York: Prometheus Books.

McCorkle, T. 1961. "Chiropractic: A Deviant Theory of Disease and Treatment in Contemporary Western Culture." *Human Organization* 20: 20–22.

McMillen, M. 2011. "Complementary and Alternative Medicine on the Rise." *WebMD*. Available at https://www.webmd.com/a-to-z-gudies/news/20110201/complementary-and-alternative-medicine-on-the-rise

Meister, A. 2010. *Evangelical Ideology in Chiropractic Medicine*. Master's Thesis, University of Pittsburgh.

National Board of Chiropractic Examiners. 2010. *Practice Analysis of Chiropractic. Chapter 1, The Chiropractic Profession*. Available at http://www.nbce.org

Paige, N. M., Miake-Lye, I. M., Booth, M. S., Beroes, J. M., Mardin, A. S., Dougherty, P., Branson, R., Tang, B., Morton, S. C. and Shekelle, P. G. 2017. "Association of Spinal Manipulative Therapy with Clinical Benefit and Harm for Acute Low Back Pain, Systematic Review and Meta-Analysis." *Journal of American Medical Association* 317(14): 1451–1460.

Roebuck, J. and B. Hunter. 1972. "The Awareness of Healthcare Quackery as Deviant Behavior." *Journal of Health and Social Behavior* 13: 162–166.

Rootman, I. and D. Mills. 1974. "Professional Behavior of American and Canadian Chiropractors." *Journal of Health and Social Behavior* 15: 3–12.

Rosenthal, S. 1986. *A Sociology of Chiropractic*. New York: Edwin Mellen.

Schneider, M. J., Evans, R., Haas, M., Leach, M., Hawk, C., Long, C., Cramer, G., Walters, O., Vihstadt, C. and Terhorst, L. 2015. U.S. Chiropractors' Attitudes, Skills and Use of Evidence-based Practice: A Cross-sectional National Survey." *Chiropractic & Manual Therapies* 23(1): 1–12.

Singh, S. and Ernst, E. 2009. *Trick or Treatment: The Undeniable Facts About Alternative Medicine*. New York: W. W. Norton and Company.

Sternberg, D. 1969. *Boys in Plight: A Case Study of Chiropractic Students Confronting a Medically-Oriented Society*. Unpublished Ph.D. Dissertation, New York University.

U.S. Department of Labor, Bureau of Labor Statistics. 2016. *Occupational Outlook Handbook 2016-2017 Edition*, Chiropractors, available at http://www.bls.gov/ooh/healthcare/chiropractors.html

Villanueva-Russell, Y. 2005. "Evidence-based Medicine and Its Implications for the Profession of Chiropractic." *Social Science & Medicine* 60(3): 545–561.

———. 2008. "An Ideal-typical Development of Chiropractic, 1895-1961: Pursuing Professional Ends Through Entrepreneurial Means." *Social Theory & Health* 6(3): 250–272.

———. 2009. "Chiropractors as Folk Devils: Published and Unpublished News Coverage of a Moral Panic." *Deviant Behavior* 30(2): 175–200.

———. 2011. "Caught in the Crosshairs: Identity and Cultural Authority within Chiropractic." *Social Science & Medicine* 72(11): 1826–1837.

Wardell, W. I. 1952. "A Marginal Professional Role: The Chiropractor." *Social Forces* 30: 33–348.

———. 1955. "The Reduction of Strain in a Marginal Social Role." *American Journal of Sociology* 61: 16–25.

———. 1961. "Public Regulation of Chiropractic." *Journal of the National Medical Association* 53: 166–172.

———. 1968. "Chiropractic Among the Healing Professions." *The ACA Journal of Chiropractic* 5: 13–19.

———. 1976. "Orthodox and Unorthodox Practitioners: Changing Relationships and the Future of Chiropractic." In R. Wallis and P. Morley (eds.), *Marginal Medicine*. New York: The Free Press, pp. 61–73.

———. 1978. "Social Factors in the Survival of Chiropractic: A Comparative View." *Sociological Symposium* 22: 6–17.

Weeks, W. B., Goertz, C. M., Meeker, W. C. and Marchiroi, D. M. 2013. "Characteristics of U.S. Adults Who Have Positive and Negative Perceptions of Doctors of Chiropractic and Chiropractic Care." *Journal of Manipulative Physiological Therapy* 39: 150–157.

Wild, P. 1978. "Social Origins and Ideology of Chiropractors: An Empirical Study of the Socialization of the Chiropractic Student." *Sociological Symposium* 22: 33–54.

Williams, S., Zipp, G. P., Cahill, T. and Parasher, R. K. 2013. "Prevalence of Burnout Among Doctors of Chiropractic in the Northeastern United States." *Journal of Manipulative Physiological Therapy* 36: 376–384.

Wong, J. 2013. "Assessing the Attitudes, Knowledge, and Perspectives of Medical Students to Chiropractic." *Journal of the Canadian Chiropractic Association* 57(1): 18–31.

Yealis, C. E., Wallace, R. B., Fisher, W. P. and R. Tolkheim. 1980. "Does Chiropractic Utilization Substitute for Less Available Medical Services?" *American Journal of Public Health* 70: 415–417.

Chapter 2

The History of Chiropractic Medicine

To begin, it is fair to say that what chiropractors do, is not new. In fact, spinal manipulation, in various forms, has been practiced for thousands of years. Healers of various types engaged in "bone setting," reduced dislocations, treated disease by manipulation, or adjusting joints. Even physicians have used manipulation techniques. Hippocrates (460–377 BCE), heralded as the father of medicine, used spinal manipulation to replace dislocated vertebrae and wrote at least three books on dealing with the treatment of bones and joints (Magner and Barrett, 1998).

Further, in the nineteenth century, there were several accounts of the use of adjustments to cure diseases. For example, Riadore (1842) wrote in *Treatise on the Irritation of the Spinal Nerves*, that without adequate blood flow, or what he termed "nervous energy," the body's ability to function was greatly impaired. Correction of this flow through the use of some forms of manipulation was said to be a key factor in a patient's overall health. Other doctors also theorized about this connection between adjusting vertebrae and healthy organs (Magner and Barrett, 1998).

As was mentioned in the previous chapter, there is real value in exploring the roots of chiropractic medicine as well as in understanding how the past has shaped the present for the profession. For some, an historical account provides a backdrop of understanding of the evolution of the profession. However, another reason to revisit chiropractic's past is to offer insight into current key issues within the profession. As we shall see, much of what chiropractic medicine has claimed as factual may have been motivated by efforts to avoid legal challenges by those providing care in the early days.

Similarly, while some will dismiss the notion of the subluxation of spinal vertebrae as part of the quackery of chiropractic, it may be that the founders of the profession stumbled upon a form of treatment but simply did not understand the fullness of its effect, nor were they very interested in proving the effectiveness of what they found. Many providers, then and today, validate chiropractic treatments by simply asking patients if they feel better. Thus the more positive responses, the greater the validation of chiropractic medicine. The reason for the initial reluctance to validate chiropractic treatments could have several sources, including the need to launch a newly established profession, to avoid legal troubles, to generate a profit for providers, or because the founders suspected some of what was being offered may have been fabricated or based on ideological and religious faith as a form of healing.

What is also interesting is that a review of the history of chiropractic is often framed differently depending upon the text in which it is found. In books that are critical of chiropractic medicine, even the historical accounts contain a condescending assessment of the events. In contrast, those manuscripts supportive of chiropractic medicine tend to portray the profession's history in light of benevolence, a resolute belief in the effectiveness of chiropractic treatment, including portraying the founders as geniuses, and as proven responses to the limits of conventional medicine. To be fair, such dichotomies are likely true of all historical accounts, but it is rather striking in the discussion of chiropractic. It is also a telling indicator of just how fragmented this profession has been from its very beginnings. That is not to say that traditional medicine does not have its own challenges, but this consistent mustang-like theme resonates throughout the entire story of the chiropractic profession.

THE EARLY BEGINNINGS OF CHIROPRACTIC MEDICINE

In perhaps one of the most important contributions to the discipline of sociology, C. Wright Mills offers a description and definition of what he terms the "sociological imagination." He says the following:

> The first fruit of this imagination—and the first lesson of the social science that embodies it—is the idea that the individual can understand his own experience and gauge his own fate only by locating himself within his period, that he can know his own chances in life only by becoming aware of those of all individuals in his circumstances. In many ways it is a terrible lesson; in many ways a magnificent one. We do not know the limits of man's capacities for supreme effort or willing degradation, for agony or glee, for pleasurable brutality or the sweetness of reason. But in our time we have come to know that the limits of

> "human nature" are frighteningly broad. We have come to know that every individual lives, from one generation to the next, in some society; that he lives out a biography, and that he lives it out within some historical sequence. By the fact of his living he contributes, however minutely, to the shaping of this society and to the course of its history, even as he is made by society and by its historical push and shove. The sociological imagination enables us to grasp history and biography and the relations between the two within society. That is its task and its promise. (Mills, 1959: 7)

Thus, Mills offers that much of our sociological understanding of groups, of people, and of the nature of social interaction can be found in the intersection between biography and history. That is, what a person believes, understands, knows, and acts upon is often a product of the time in history they have lived, their particular family of origin, and their individual experiences and interactions with others. The understanding of the person, how they see the world, how they act in it, and their particular point of view on a variety of topics are based on these factors (Mills, 1959).

This context of understanding and appreciation of the people involved applies to the development of chiropractic medicine as well. It is a relatively simple matter to chronicle the starting date and founding father of chiropractic medicine; a simple Internet search can provide the details and the timeline for the development of the profession. This is important information and it will be offered in this chapter. However, a much greater appreciation of the development of chiropractic medicine is achieved if we can understand how and under what circumstances the field developed. This context of understanding is crucial to gaining sufficient insight into the current state of affairs within the profession.

In other words, it is one thing to suggest that the founding father of chiropractic, Daniel David (D. D.) Palmer, was a genius who created chiropractic medicine out of his own creative thoughts. While debate can occur over the accuracy of such a statement, it is much more valuable to understand that intersection between biography and history, to know more about Palmer's upbringing, where he lived, what were the circumstances of his social development, along with the state of how people viewed medicine during that particular point in history.

That information provides a much more comprehensive understanding of the development of chiropractic medicine than a simple listing of dates, times, and events. It also helps to understand the strong religious influence of chiropractic medicine and extends the understanding of the field in a way that goes beyond attributing it to a particular person. What follows is an assessment of the facts in light of the framework Mills identified as essential to our understanding of chiropractic medicine.

Intersection: Biography

Daniel David Palmer was born on March 7, 1845, in Brown's Corner, Ontario, just east of Toronto. Palmer's father, Thomas, believed in the religious teachings offered by Seventh Day Adventists, who took the instructions of the Bible literally, and who believed in living a disciplined and righteous life. Adventism was one of many popular religious movements at the time in the United States and was part of a larger religious movement in the nineteenth century. At its base, this movement, sometimes referred to as *religious revivalism*, stressed a personal relationship with God along with a spiritual conversion that launched such a connection. D. D. Palmer grew up in this type of environment, in which many families were poor and did not place a great deal of emphasis on education. In fact, Palmer received a formal education only until about the age of eleven (Harrison, 1995).

In 1865, the elder Palmer moved his family to Iowa in the hopes of better job opportunities, as the Civil War had ended and Reconstruction began. As an adult, D. D. Palmer operated a wide range of businesses, from raising bees to growing fruit, to operating a grocery store. By 1881, his third wife died leaving Palmer to care for two daughters, aged eight and six from his second marriage, and a son, Bartlett Joshua (B. J.) Palmer, who would eventually become the most popular figure in the history of chiropractic medicine. The relationship between Palmer and his son was a difficult one, as was the son's relationship with his stepmothers. This tension would ultimately result in a permanent estrangement between father and son (Benedetti and MacPhail, 2002).

At about the same time, spiritualism and magnetic healing became topics of interest for Palmer. Spiritualists believe that it was possible to talk to the dead through mystical means, most notably the séance. Magnetic healers believed they could treat a variety of illnesses by diverting and clearing the way for *animal magnetism*, a term used to describe the universal flow of life, which flowed through the body like a liquid. Healers were said to be able to clear the blockages and allow the natural flow to resume, which allowed the body to remain healthy (Mesmer, 1779).

In the 1880s, magnetic healing mixed with a form of religious revivalism, especially in rural areas of the country, was said to cure a variety of illnesses. The most well-known magnetic healer at the time was Franz Mesmer, who was popular around the late 1700s. Mesmer was a German physician who believed that the universe was filled with fluid. He wrote, for example, that the spaces between the grains of sand could be filled with water and the spaces in water could be filled with air. Even spaces within the air were permeated with invisible ether. When the latter was present in a living thing, he called it *animal magnetism*. Mesmer believed that disease was the result of blockages of the universal fluid, or animal magnetism, in the body. The blockages dilated the blood vessels which inhibited the body's ability to thrive and heal itself. In contrast, a body that had sufficient animal magnetism would not become ill. More broadly, this notion of animal magnetism was linked philosophically to *Vitalism,* which asserts that life is driven by an invisible spiritual force.

Mesmer practiced magnetic healing in Vienna and his charisma and flamboyance convinced many patients that his treatments were effective, particularly wealthy women. However, physicians quickly took exception to what amounted to questionable treatments and labeled Mesmer a fraud. While his early success eventually led to a decline in popularity in Europe, it made a significant impact in America (Harrison, 1995; Mesmer, 1888).

As late as the 1880s, magnetic healing was still a popular treatment for many illnesses. Palmer took courses from Paul Caster, the leading proponent of magnetic healing at the time, and became a doctor of magnetic healing (Harrison, 1995). In 1886, Palmer opened an office in a small town in Iowa, near the Mississippi River. However, he found that there were other healers who competed for his patients, which made it difficult for him to sustain his practice. About a year later he opened a new office in Davenport, Iowa, and the lack of competition in the area resulted in much greater success (Benedetti and MacPhail, 2002).

Palmer advertised as a doctor who did not need surgery or drugs to cure illnesses. Like Mesmer, he treated patients by placing one hand under the problem area and the other above it so that "magnetic radiation" could flow from one hand to the other. Unlike other magnetic healers, who took a more comprehensive approach to healing the entire body, Palmer claimed to be able to isolate the problem and concentrate his magnetic healing into a focused area. This claim, along with some shrewd advertising, resulted in a successful practice, attracting patients from other parts of the state and even the entire country (Benedetti and Macphail, 2002). Palmer's claims of no drugs and no surgery were important to this success, particularly given the way medicine was perceived by the public during this period.

Intersection: Medicine During this Era

As many historians have noted, the post–Civil War era was a turbulent time for the United States, socially, economically, religiously, and particularly in the development of medicine (Foner, 2015). From a spiritual perspective, American Protestant religions had already passed through two "Great Awakenings" of religious passion. While Calvinists were largely responsible for the first experience with this movement in the Northeast, the second Great Awakening, from about 1790 to 1830, occurred in the South. These revivals and dramatic exhortations of the Gospel, sometimes known as *fire and brimstone sermons*, had a strong emotional content rather than an intellectual appeal to the Bible (Scott, 2000).

By the end of the Civil War, emotionally charged religious beliefs created newer movements, such as the development of Pentacostal, Fundamentalism, and Adventists efforts, which focused on the imminent return of Jesus Christ and the need for a religious conversion of being "born again" through a spiritual epiphany for practitioners. These religious movements were also heavily influenced by the development of modernity, and a movement sometimes referred to as *American Romanticism* (Scott, 2000).

This era was characterized by a rejection of science and intellectualism, brought on by a reaction to the Industrial Revolution and the Age of Enlightenment of the eighteenth century. It focused on a celebration of the common man's experience with nature and emphasized getting in touch with one's emotions rather than Man's reasoning ability. The notion of truth was questioned as a social construct and seen as inherently subjective. This movement, which could be seen as an early version of the Hippie movement of the 1960s and 1970s, was not bound to the rigors of science and empirical inquiry, and focused more on rejecting all that was connected to industrialization (Scott, 2000; Friebert et al., 1994).

American Romanticism influenced literature, politics, music, arts, and people's thinking about medicine. The election of Andrew Jackson as president in 1829, who prided himself as an advocate for the common man, who had a disdain for the ruling aristocracy of the past, resonated with the American people. The combined effect of Romanticism and Jacksonian democracy during this period produced some unique American traits, including religious evangelism (King, 1992; Friebert et al., 1994).

In literature, the American Romanticism movement was personified in the popular works of writers such as Emerson, Hawthorne, and Melville, and consistent with its view of the world, was less interested in science and religious proscriptions, such as the tenets of Calvinism (Woodlief, 2012). These writers, who were responding to the changing social and political landscape, often told stories that called attention to the inequalities found in American democracy. Thus, the clash between the reality and the idealism of the times resulted in writers of this era creating stories that championed individualism in a fragmented society (Woodlief, 2012).

Thus, American Romanticism consisted of a general theme of mistrust of science during this time, and of the intellectuals who espoused it. The most noted target of this suspicion were doctors. Unfortunately, at the time, medicine was not fully developed and knowledge about illnesses and curing diseases was really in its infancy. This understanding, of course, did little to enhance the public's trust of physicians. For example, at the beginning of the nineteenth century, most doctors believed that all disease resulted from the overstimulation of nerves and blood (Friebert et al., 1994).

To address these problems, doctors practiced what has come to be known as *heroic medicine*. This included bleeding patients, creating blisters on the skin, and administering laxatives. Heroic medicine was painful and ineffective. Naturally, these features made it widely unpopular with patients. Until the 1840s, the only anesthetics available were alcohol and opium and doctors had little understanding of germ theory or of how to avoid spreading infection. Despite these challenges, heroic medicine continued to be widely practiced by physicians, largely because it was all that was known at the time (King, 1982; Friebert et al., 1994; Benedetti and MacPhail, 2002).

While some progressive physicians in the United States began stressing the use of data and clinical examination as part of their overall treatment, the lack of understanding of basic principles about bacteria and infection had a host of consequences for patients. Surgery, during this period of American history, was particularly challenging. At the beginning of the Civil War, for example, for every soldier who died in battle, two died from dysentery, diarrhea, typhoid, or malaria (Civilwarhome.com). A total of 560,000 soldiers on both sides died from diseases and an additional 200,000 died from battlefield injuries, often postoperative infections. There was no antiseptic surgery at the time. When doctors encountered a massive battle wound, the most frequent solution was amputation (Civilwarhome.com).

While there were significant advances in medicine as a result of the Civil War, including research notes on disease and the treatment of wounds, the public's perception of doctors remained quite negative (King, 1982; Friebert et al., 1994; Benedetti and MacPhail, 2002). The poor reputation of physicians during this period was underscored by their lack of adequate training. In the early parts of the nineteenth century, students had to purchase tickets to attend lectures in medical school, medical students were often illiterate, and some even had to bring their own cadavers for dissection if their medical school could not provide a sufficient number (Benedetti and MacPhail, 2002). By 1875, there were seventy-five medical schools throughout the country, but these were small and proprietary, and had no standard curriculum along with relaxed entrance exams. As one commentator noted, medical education was little more than an apprenticeship during this period (Benedetti and MacPhail, 2002).

By the middle of the century, enormous strides were made in medicine and in science. In Europe, there were discoveries made by Pasteur about germ theory, along with those made by Lister, who had developed the concept of communicable diseases and bacteria, but the germ theory was still not a part of the American model of medicine. It was not until 1880 that Dr. William Mayo first practiced antiseptic surgery in Rochester, Minnesota. The discoveries in science brought with them a number of developments in medical treatment, including vaccination and antibiotics. Consequently, there were dramatic decreases in mortality and the average life span saw improvement (Simpson, 2012).

As a result, the medical profession's standing improved somewhat. By the end of the century, efforts were also made to reevaluate the state of medical education in this country. The Flexner Report, a study that examined the state of medical education in the United States, was instrumental in changes in how physicians practiced and began using science and evidence-based techniques. In fact, by 1930, only 76 of the 168 medical schools remained open and the number of medical school graduates decreased from more than 5,000 per year to 3,636. The Flexner Report also targeted chiropractors, who were referred to as "unconscionable quacks who should be dealt with by the public prosecutor and grand jury." This strongly worded statement resulted in the AMA, whose Medical Education Committee promoted the Flexner Report, to consider how to respond to the chiropractic profession (Flexner, 1910).

However, while these discoveries and changes were paramount to the development of medicine, the public's image and understanding of the profession remained skeptical and negative. People were still concerned about illnesses and looked to other means to solve their problems without surgery, drugs, or concerns about infection. It makes sense, then, that the natural medicine movement of the 1880s was in part a product of the fears about medicine, along with the strong influence of religious fundamentalism.

The dubious practices and disregard for logic or reasonableness when it came to health crazes was the backdrop to D. D. Palmer's ideas about healing and illness. The Popular Health Movement was characterized by a return to nature, with fresh air, clean water, exercise, good nutrition, and the use of natural herbs to cure illnesses. In response, the medical profession dismissed this movement as cultism (Friebert et al., 1994).

Sometimes referred to the "golden age of quackery" a wide range of cures developed to address an assortment of ailments. It was the era of the traveling circus, medicine shows, and snake oil salesmen, who believed they had whatever cure the public needed. Hydrotherapists, for example, claimed that injecting patients with water or wrapping them in wet blankets was a cure for a variety of illnesses. Patent medicines developed, which were shrewdly marketed to the public, and were wildly successful. According to one estimate, quack medicines were generating over $3 million in sales by 1859 and $75 million by 1904 (Benedetti and MacPhail, 2002).

Thus, what Palmer was offering was similar to what many others were presenting to a disenchanted public: a chance to avoid being treated by doctors, who were viewed with suspicion and whose competence was questioned. This was particularly appealing if the natural healers could present their treatments in a religious context. The religious component, coupled with a mistrust of science and of medicine, created a host of profitable opportunities for providers.

It is a bit ironic that these natural healers had less training than physicians and whose motives were likely generating profit more than divine inspiration, but the public flocked to these questionable treatments without any meaningful examination of their effectiveness. The reason, as was mentioned, is likely linked to the social themes of the times: religious revivalism, a distrust of science, and a desire to be at one with nature. This is why so many of the elixirs that were created were touted as being all-natural and comprised of vegetables, herbs, and other extracts (Friebert et al., 1994).

Thus, when Palmer opened his clinic in Davenport, Iowa, there was not anything particularly noteworthy about what he offered in the way of treatment, although his location may have proved to be a successful one. Rather, Palmer's magnetic treatments were one of several popular solutions to medical problems for people of that time period. As is often the case with important discoveries, happenstance played a role in the development of chiropractic medicine. It was a chance encounter with a janitor in the building Palmer was leasing that was the landmark event in Palmer's life. As he describes it,

> Harvey Lillard, a janitor in the Ryan Block, where I had my office, had been so deaf for 17 years that he could not hear the racket of a wagon on the street or the ticking of a watch. I made inquiry as to the cause of his deafness and was informed that when he was exerting himself in a cramped, stooped position, he felt something give way in his back and immediately became deaf. An examination showed a vertebra racked from its normal position. I reasoned that if that vertebra was replaced, the man's hearing should be restored. With this object in view, a half-hour's talk persuaded Mr. Lillard to allow me to replace it. I racked it into position by using the spinous process as a lever and soon the man could hear as before. There was nothing "accidental" about this, as it was accomplished with an object in view and the result expected was obtained. There was nothing "crude" about this adjustment; it was specific, so much so that no Chiropractor has equaled it. (Palmer, 1910)

Palmer later stated he treated another patient for what he described as "heart trouble." He adjusted this patient's vertebrae and it produced relief. As a result, Palmer believed he had been given the explanation for the cause of 95 percent of all disease. That is, bones out of place put pressure on the blood vessels and nerves and this caused illness and weakness in the body. By adjusting these misplaced bones, chiropractors could offer effective treatment. Palmer later called the misalignments *luxations* or dislocations. Ultimately, Palmer referred to these problems as *subluxations*, as they were less than a full dislocation of the vertebrae (Palmer, 1910). In 1896 with the help of a local minister, Palmer coined the term *chiropractic* from the Greek words meaning "done by hand" to describe his newly created form of treatment, one that was distinguished from all others (Simpson, 2012).

The account offered by Palmer of how chiropractic medicine was created has several versions in the literature. In one telling, Palmer was listening to Lillard recount a joke and in response, Palmer good-naturedly slapped Lillard on the back with a book. In response, Lillard began to realize a slight improvement in his hearing. There are also questions about which vertebrae Palmer adjusted and even the date of the event has been questioned. While there may be a bit of legend construction at work (Wardell, 1950), and while some even doubted that Palmer performed the first adjustment (osteopaths claimed that they were the first to have discovered misaligned vertebrae as a cause of disease in 1874), Palmer claimed his treatments were far superior to anything anyone else had ever performed. Palmer also argued that osteopaths were focused on the free flowing of health to occur, whereas he was more concerned with reducing what he described as friction and inflammation as the main source of illness (Palmer, 1910).

Over the next decade, Palmer revised his thinking about chiropractic medicine and began to further distance it from osteopathic medicine. However, Palmer was rather circumspect with sharing his discoveries about illness as well as his techniques to treat them. Later, Palmer began teaching his method to his son, B. J., and to a select number of students. However, their training consisted of observing Palmer as he treated patients, which took, on average, about thirty seconds. There were no textbooks, lectures, notes, patient records, or charts (Wardell, 1992). It appeared from some accounts, to resemble how doctors were trained in medicine at the time—as apprenticeships, but without any meaningful direction. Such an approach created opportunities for students to have their own interpretations of what constituted chiropractic treatments and their own explanations of what was occurring.

One student in particular, Oakley Smith, eventually opened his own chiropractic school, the American School of Chiropractic. While Palmer also established his own Palmer School of Chiropractic, from the very beginning there were questions about various interpretations of Palmer's original techniques and many of the new schools had their own ideas about treatments and other forms of therapy. Palmer referred to those schools who blended his techniques with other treatments "Mixers" (Palmer, 1910).

Palmer maintained that his was the only true version of chiropractic, which he referred to as "Straight" chiropractic. This distinction, along with newer versions of what types of treatments chiropractors should perform, remains evident today. Straight chiropractors believe their focus should be only on addressing subluxations and allowing the body to heal itself. Mixers still believe that some illnesses are a result of misalignments of the spine, but are much more likely to refer patients to medical doctors for certain ailments (Keating, 1995). Both groups believed in the idea of the vertebrae subluxation, a topic we will be returning to in subsequent chapters, as it relates to chiropractic's scope of practice and philosophy of treatment.

Palmer refined his theory of chiropractic in subsequent years, focusing primarily on nerves. Palmer eventually believed that there were two types of nerves, those that control the voluntary motion of the body and those that were responsible for involuntary actions, such as digestion. These latter forms were called *Innate* (Palmer, 1910). This latter phrase is critical to understanding some of the versions of chiropractic medicine that exist today.

Palmer began to think of "Innate" not simply as a way to describe involuntary nerves, but as a form of higher intelligence that controlled the function of the body. Palmer, writing as late as 1906, wrote that almost all bodily functions are managed by Innate, except where those nerves are interfered with, which causes abnormal functioning in the body. This is a critical development in the history of chiropractic since it places much greater emphasis on the nerves and on a form of spiritual healing (the universal force in the world that flows through the body). Thus, the Innate normally allows the body to heal itself in most circumstances because innate intelligence is a part of the much larger universal intelligence in the world. However, as Palmer pointed out, subluxations block the flow of Innate by pinching or impeding the nerves in the spine (Benedetti and MacPhail, 2002).

About four years later, Palmer again revised his thinking about the pinching of nerves. In 1910, Palmer believed that a body's health depended on the state of what he called its *Tone*. Tone was said to be delivered to the body through the nerves and its source was innate intelligence. If misaligned joints inhibited the nerves, there would be an increase or decrease of tension in the nerve. Similar to guitar strings that needed to be maintained at the proper tension so they could remain in proper tune, nerves with adequate tension allow the body to maintain optimum health—and only chiropractors were sufficiently trained to understand how to properly tune those nerves (Magner and Barrett, 1998).

The impact of this thinking was significant: subluxations caused an increase in nerve tension and that resulted in excessive nerve vibration. This vibration heated the blood and the excess heat could cause inflammation, kill tissue, and stop organs from functioning. Infections, fevers, swelling, and other problems were not the result of germs, but a result of nerves that became too active as a result of bones becoming misaligned in the body (Palmer, 1909).

But the story does not end there. Recall Palmer's deeply held religious beliefs. These now came back into play in his understanding of chiropractic medicine. Palmer became more convinced that the creation of universal intelligence, which perpetuated the universe, was God. Palmer took some of the lessons from Mesmer's magnetism theories and integrated it with his own deeply held religious beliefs. He believed that the innate intelligence was a part of everyone and the Innate wanted to "communicate" with chiropractors, who were the designated healers that fostered the body's ability to heal itself. Palmer also believed that the secret of chiropractic was sent to him directly by God (Simpson, 2012; Benedetti and MacPhail, 2002).

By 1910, Palmer had returned to the religious beliefs he embraced prior to the discovery of chiropractic. He believed that chiropractors did not treat diseases, they simply listened to the Innate and used their hands to allow it to manifest itself in the body. As a type of Messiah, Palmer also felt that he was the only one who could impart this combination of philosophy, art, and science in his new form of treatment, chiropractic (Benedetti and MacPhail, 2002).

Part of the interpretation for Palmer's sudden departure from science and his early thoughts about chiropractic into a form of religion was likely due to the legal challenges that the profession was facing at the time. It was also the case that new chiropractic schools were espousing many of the techniques and theories Palmer had developed years earlier. The success of some of these schools, particularly due to B. J. Palmer's efforts, may have been perceived as threatening to Palmer, who claimed to be the only one who was divinely provided with the key to chiropractic medicine. More than likely, however, were Palmer's concerns about legal threats from the medical profession. Palmer had already been jailed for practicing medicine without a license and other chiropractors had received similar sanctions (Manger and Barrett, 1998).

Perhaps in an effort to thwart the legal charges against chiropractors, Palmer felt the need to separate chiropractic from traditional medicine in a dramatic way. This is speculation, of course, but the fallout from such a strategy has many far-reaching implications. It is not the case, as many experts have noted, that Palmer wanted chiropractic to be seen as a form of religion, although his own beliefs surely influenced his understanding of the profession (Magner and Barrett, 1998). Rather, he is said to have wanted some protection from the external attacks from others who claimed chiropractors were engaging in the unlawful and unethical treatment of patients (Palmer, 1914).

In sum, Palmer's ideas about chiropractic medicine had little philosophy and no science. He was heavily influenced by spiritual ideas, even going so far as to claim that the idea for chiropractic was a message from God, and borrowed concepts from osteopathy and mesmerism. The many revisions of this theory, coupled with his lack of scientific validation, have continued to plague the profession (Benedetti and MacPhail, 2002). In 1913, Palmer died of typhoid fever at the age of sixty-eight.

B. J. Palmer's Intersection Between Biography and History

Another key figure in the development of chiropractic medicine was Palmer's son, B. J. Palmer. B. J.'s relationship with his father was an acrimonious one. Like his father and many people during that era, B. J. had only a limited formal education. Descriptions of his childhood, particularly with his many stepmothers (Palmer was married multiple times over the course of his life), were said to be filled with neglect and abuse. By his own description, B. J. once testified at a trial that he was kicked out of his home at the age of eleven and forced to live on the streets. His experiences with homelessness and hustling activities led to brief episodes in jail as a young man, along with an exposure to the seedier side of life. In 1898, B. J. ran away and joined the circus. For three years, Palmer's exposure to the showmanship of circus life provided good training for what was to come later as he assumed control of chiropractic medicine (Keating, 1995; Magner and Barrett, 1998).

In 1901 B. J. returned to Davenport and graduated from his father's chiropractic school. A short time later, after D. D. Palmer left Davenport, B. J. found himself in control of his father's clinic and school, which was awash in debt. With the help of a local businessman and some crafty advertising, B. J. was able to restore the clinic as a profitable business venture. When D. D. returned to Davenport a few years later, the chiropractic college was barely surviving and the Palmers and other chiropractors were under a threat of legal action against them for practicing medicine without a license (Keating, 1995; Benedetti and McPhail, 2002).

While his relationship with his father was always a tense one, with many disagreements and arguments, D. D. Palmer's conviction and jail sentence was a watershed event—B. J. refused to let him back to the Palmer College campus. The event resulted in D. D. selling his share of the College to B. J. and led to his departure from Davenport. D. D. moved on to Oklahoma and Oregon where he opened other chiropractic schools. His lack of success with these ventures ultimately led to a return to Davenport in 1913. Two months later, D. D. died of typhoid fever (Keating, 1995; Magner and Barrett, 1998).

As a gifted speaker and salesman, B. J. attracted a following of students. He also made every effort to distinguish chiropractic from medicine and osteopathy. His lack of understanding of science and basic anatomy did not prevent him from using his marketing skills to establish chiropractic as a disease-curing, all-encompassing method of healing. Nor did it keep him from modifying chiropractic philosophies and techniques as the need arose (Keating, 1992).

In the early 1930s, for example, B. J. declared that only the topmost spinal bones should be manipulated and the rest of the spine would "fall into place." Ever the advertiser, B. J. gave this new technique, which was incongruent with what was taught at chiropractic colleges, including Palmer's, the name H. I. O., which stood for "hole in one." In other words, if the chiropractor made this adjustment, the patient would be healed—one technique, one cure. Chiropractors had been taught that misaligned vertebrae occurred throughout the spine and this caused certain diseases and specific adjustments cured those ailments. Palmer's new theory rejected this idea and suggested that chiropractors were using incorrect treatments on patients and needed additional training in this new technique (Homola and Barrett, 1999).

These changes and events occurred while many chiropractors were being arrested and jailed for practicing medicine without a license. In response, in 1905, B. J. Palmer created the Universal Chiropractor's Association to provide some level of legal protection for chiropractors who faced these types of allegations. Little did he realize that a landmark case would be presented to this newly established group a year later (Benedetti and MacPhail, 2002).

In 1907, Shegataro Morikubo, a student of Palmer's, had graduated in 1906 and opened a practice in La Crosse, Wisconsin. Morikubo was charged with practicing medicine and osteopathy without a license. The attorney for Morikubo, Tom Morris, was able to convince the prosecutor to drop the charge of practicing medicine without a license, but the charge of practicing osteopathy without one remained. In an effort to craft a defense against this charge, Morris argued that chiropractors focused on the impingement of nerves, whereas osteopaths focused on the role of blockages of blood flow in all joints of the body (Benedetti and MacPhail, 2002).

Although Morris convinced the prosecution that chiropractors were distinctive from osteopaths, in that chiropractors only focused on the nerves of the spine, many chiropractors, particularly those who espoused Palmer's original ideas, believed that misalignments of the spine could cause impingements on the nerve as well as restricting blood flow. Some historical accounts of this trial suggest that both Morris and B. J. Palmer knew they were being less than honest about this explanation, but the argument was a convincing one. Moreover, as an additional effort to distinguish chiropractic from other types of medicine, a new set of terminology for the techniques of chiropractic emerged as a result of this trial. Thus, the language used and the narrative about chiropractic medicine shifted, not because of a reassessment of the treatments, but purely as a means to avoid prosecution and legal disputes (Benedetti and MacPhail, 2002).

By all accounts, B. J. Palmer was charismatic and articulate, and had a shrewd sense of marketing and showmanship. A compelling storyteller, students and chiropractors alike were enamored with his vision for the field as well as his promises of wild success. Evidence of this is seen in enrollments in the Palmer School of Chiropractic, which rose from about 400 students in 1904 to about 2,800 in 1921. Some of that increase was undoubtedly the result of men returning from World War I with government funding for their education, but a part of it has to be attributed to Palmer's influence (Benedetti and MacPhail, 2002).

One of the ways through which B. J. Palmer was able to sustain the chiropractic school and spread the word about chiropractic was his purchase of a small AM radio station. Because of the location of the station's antenna, people from a sizable portion of the United States and Canada heard Palmer's message. Fortuitously, the purchase of the station came at a time when the popularity of radio was just beginning. In addition to the news and entertainment, Palmer made sure the listening audience received a regular dose of information on chiropractic medicine, as sponsors of particular radio shows, as advertisements, and even as lectures from the Palmer College of Chiropractic (Keating, 1995).

In fact, some observers note that Palmer had a corner on the chiropractic education market as well. He owned the chiropractic printing and merchandising business and his summer lecture series attracted thousands of chiropractors from all over the world. It seemed like he could do no wrong when it came to promoting and marketing the profession. However, perhaps it was greed, perhaps due to a belief that he could not fail, or perhaps both, Palmer made a crucial mistake in 1924, one that would resonate within the profession for decades. In fact, this decision not only raised questions about Palmer's role as the undisputed leader of chiropractic, but many began to question his trustworthiness as well. This event also served to further divide the profession (Keating, 1995).

In 1924, while presiding over one of his annual Lycenum and conference in Davenport, Palmer introduced what he contended was the most important technological invention in chiropractic history: the Neurocalometer. This instrument was said to allow chiropractors to easily and accurately locate subluxations. The instrument had two narrowly spaced probes that could register a difference in temperature between them. Dossa Evins, the inventor, believed the Neurocalometer would allow chiropractors to easily identify subluxations since the nerve impulse blockages that are created with a subluxation also created changes in skin temperature. If that were true, then the Neurocalometer could easily identify the location of a subluxation. Palmer felt that the Neurocalometer was the solution to bringing chiropractic back to its fundamental roots (Benedetti and MacPhail, 2012; Keating, 1991; Newborg, 2010).

Palmer told the audience that this device would only be available to straight chiropractors and only on a leased basis for ten years; one could not purchase it. Despite the lack of evidence of its effectiveness, and despite the exorbitant costs of leasing the device, at a cost of nearly $2,200 (the price of a home during that time period), over a thousand were leased in the first year and another thousand were leased the year after. But while some bought into the ploy, many other chiropractors disagreed, particularly because of the draconian measures used by Palmer in making the Neurocalometer available to them. This resulted in a split within the profession and damaged Palmer's standing within the chiropractic community (Keating, 1992).

The introduction of the Neurocalmeter resulted in several faculty members at the Palmer College resigning in protest and forming their own chiropractic college. This had a negative impact on enrollment at the Palmer College. The introduction of the Great Depression severely impacted the College as well; in fact, the Palmer College went into bankruptcy during the Depression. Were it not for the support from the radio station, the Palmer School of Chiropractic would have been completely disbanded (Magner and Barrett, 1998).

The failure of the Neurocalometer, along with its unsubstantiated advertising claims, dubious modifications in techniques to force chiropractors to pay for additional training, and the outlandish claims made by Palmer about chiropractic medicine, all had a significant impact on the profession. By all accounts, Palmer did not believe in research; rather he attempted to reduce chiropractic to simple non-scientific principles at a time when the profession had no response to a society that demanded proof that chiropractic worked (Wardell, 1992).

For all of his claims of legitimacy in chiropractic medicine being the cure of all disease, most historical accounts show that B. J. made use of traditional medicine when he was ill, although this was not done publicly. B. J. developed colon cancer and sought traditional medical treatment as a result. Ultimately, he died of the disease in 1961 at the age of seventy-nine (Magner and Barrett, 1998).

LICENSURE AND LEGITIMACY FOR CHIROPRACTIC

The *Morikubo* case provided some comfort to chiropractors since it allowed them to continue practicing without fear of prosecution. However, the lessons learned from this case demonstrated the need for chiropractors to gain some level of validity and credibility by using the political and legal system to require licenses to practice, similar to physicians. This, many chiropractors felt, would give chiropractic medicine a legitimate standing as a profession.

The limited understanding of medicine during this period, along with concerns about chiropractors operating unsupervised, led thirty-two states to pass licensure laws by 1925. In some cases, when such laws were passed, chiropractors who did not want to pay for licensure or to have their practices regulated either closed their businesses or simply moved to a state that did not have licensure laws. In other instances, chiropractors redefined the treatments they offered, such as arguing they provided physiotherapy, which did not require a license (Magner and Barrett, 1998).

While many legislators were concerned about chiropractors' use of the law as a protection from science, some believed that the laws could provide a mechanism of social control over the profession. In many states, the biggest obstacle to licensure were chiropractors themselves. Disagreements about the scope of practice and the proper nature of chiropractic treatments often led to delays in the passing of legislation. In the end, those factions within chiropractic that were able to marshal greater political influence often had their version of chiropractic written into law. This diversity is seen even today as each state dictates the scope of practice for its chiropractors and there is wide variation in what that scope entails. Some states allow chiropractors to perform gynecological exams, and do anything short of surgery, while other states allow chiropractors to prescribe certain forms of medicine to patients. In contrast, some states narrowly limit the scope of practice for chiropractors to only treating neck and back injuries (Dynamic Chiropractic, 2014).

Along with the discussions about licensure, many states began to recognize that if they were allowing chiropractors to perform a variety of treatments on patients that were similar to physicians, it was reasonable that chiropractors should be able to demonstrate some level of competency in those areas. While many chiropractors did not wish to be held to such standards, by the late 1950s many states established basic science boards to conduct examinations on chiropractic students to make sure they met certain guidelines of understanding.

By 1959, twenty-four states required chiropractors to successfully pass these tests, the same ones for medical and osteopathic licensure. The problem was that a majority of chiropractic graduates were not able to complete the exams successfully. According to one historian, between 1927 and 1953, about 86 percent of medical students and only 23 percent of the 2,500 chiropractic students passed (Rosenthal, 1986). In Nebraska, no chiropractor passed the exam between 1929 and 1950. The problem was that since it was not a nationwide requirement, those chiropractors who failed the exam either moved to a state where the exam was not required or practiced without a license (Rosenthal, 1986; Magner and Barrett, 1998).

Clearly the competency exam idea had merit, but as a practical and political matter, efforts were made to revise the exams in such a way to focus on what chiropractors actually did rather than asking them to understand all aspects of medicine. These revisions restricted the content of the exams to areas of the spine and by 1979, these exams were repealed completely. Today, chiropractic students must pass tests in basic sciences, along with several other practical exams to demonstrate their competency in diagnosing and treating patients (American Chiropractic Association, 2017).

As was mentioned, the *Morikubo* case resulted in the realization that chiropractors needed to have some level of unification or a collective voice if it was to respond effectively to challenges from other professions. Thus, as a form of protection from lawsuits as well as to influence legislation about licensure and training, chiropractic organizations were formed in the early 1920s. The immediate problem, of course, were the internal disagreements about chiropractic medicine and their differing philosophies. As a result, many organizations were formed.

For instance, the American Chiropractic Association was created in the 1920s and has as its roots the National Chiropractic Association. It states on its website that its vision is, in part,

- Collaboration with other health care disciplines and integration into all health care delivery models that enhance individual health, public health, wellness, and safety.
- Change in public policy, and legislative and regulatory arenas, resulting in a more effective U.S. health care system.
- Improvement in health care access and freedom of choice of heath care providers for the American people, without discriminatory obstacles.
- Increased value of health care for patients, policymakers, and the public through the high professional and educational standards of the chiropractic profession (acatoday.org).

The tone and content of the website suggest that this organization is taking a broad-based view of the role of chiropractic in medicine and how it might work seamlessly with traditional medicine while maintaining its own identity and purpose.

The International Chiropractic Association (ICA) has its roots in B. J. Palmer's Chiropractic Health Bureau. It states its objectives, in part, as the following:

- Maintain and promote chiropractic's unique identity as a non-therapeutic, drugless, and surgical free health science based on its fundamental principles and philosophy.
- Work harmoniously with other health care organizations and governments in a global humanitarian effort to foster chiropractic and spinal hygiene in the fields of family health (including children, women and the elderly), and occupational health.
- Work for full inclusion of chiropractic in all public and private health care delivery programs.
- Foster the professional and technical development of the Doctor of Chiropractic through programs of continuing education, research, political and social action (chiropractic.org).

Notice the language here suggests a concerted effort to legitimize the profession and a theme of advocacy and credibility. This group has also identified where they stand on a number of critical issues within the profession, such as maintenance care, the treatment of children, and other issues. While virtually all the groups discuss the need for collaboration with other health care providers, along with the notion that the ultimate goal is the welfare and health of the patient, some organizations are clearly more involved in promoting an agenda than others.

The Federation of Straight Chiropractors and Organizations (FSCO) was created in 1976 and consists of an extreme version of straight chiropractors. On its website, one phrase adequately captures their identity, purpose and mission. It reads "Vertebral Subluxation Correction . . . Nothing More . . . Nothing Less . . . Nothing Else" (ifcochiro.org).

The World Chiropractic Alliance (WCA), created in 1989, describes itself as a not-for-profit organization that serves as the voice of conservative straight chiropractors. They claim to be the only major chiropractic organization that defends its philosophical and vitalistic foundations and believes that adjustments should begin at birth and continue throughout a person's life, regardless of whether they exhibit any back or neck pain.

The WCA does not believe in vaccinations because they contend that chiropractic adjustments correct any deficiencies in one's immune system. They state, as their major premise, that there is a universal intelligence in all matter and continually gives to all its properties and actions, thus maintaining it in existence. What they call the secondary principles include the following:

- The expression of this intelligence through matter is the chiropractic meaning of life.
- Life is a Triune, having three necessary united factors, namely, Intelligence, Force, and Matter.

- In order to have 100% life, there must be 100% Intelligence, 100% Force, 100% Matter.
- A living thing has an inborn intelligence within its body, called Innate Intelligence.
- There can be interference with the transmission of Innate Forces, which causes dis-ease (worldchiropracticalliance.org).

The National Association of Chiropractic Medicine (NACM) began in 1984. It describes itself as: "a consumer advocacy association of chiropractors who confine their scope of practice to scientific parameters and seek to make legitimate the utilization of professional manipulative procedures in mainstream health care delivery." The NACM offers consumer assistance in finding member practitioners (Chiromed.org).

The World Federation of Chiropractic Medicine (WFCM) was established in Sydney, Australia, in 1988 and represents eighty-eight countries. Its goals, according to their website, are to

- promote uniform high standards of chiropractic education, research, and practice;
- develop an informed public opinion among all peoples with respect to chiropractic;
- uniting members of the chiropractic profession and protecting the character and status of the profession;
- acting with national and international organizations to provide information and other assistance in the fields of chiropractic and world health (wfc.org).

There are many other organizations that are part of the chiropractic profession, but these are the most widely known or have the largest membership lists. As we will discuss in subsequent chapters, each group appears to have its own ideas about the role of chiropractic medicine, with some taking a more international focus, while others narrowly define what the role of chiropractic should be in treating patients, and others seem to be offering a much broader vision for the profession. These are important considerations because such sharp disagreements continue to have a deleterious impact on the profession in the minds of others, particularly in medicine.

PHYSICIANS VERSUS CHIROPRACTORS—THE AMA

In 1961, in response to the growing concern about chiropractic medicine, the AMA created a committee on quackery, whose mission was to contain and eliminate the chiropractic profession. In 1966, the *Journal of the American*

Medical Association published a report, based on the catalogs from each of the thirteen chiropractic schools around the country, particularly those approved by chiropractic organizations. Only about half of the faculty listed in these catalogs had recognized academic degrees, and while some faculty claimed degrees from accredited schools, records of their credentials could not be found. The report also found that many of the faculty who taught basic science courses did not have a degree in the subjects they were teaching (American Medical Association, 1966).

In the 1960s the AMA's committee on quackery sponsored conferences, helped prepare publications, and engaged in other activities intended to discourage doctors from professionally associating with chiropractors. In 1966, the AMA's House of Delegates passed a resolution calling chiropractic an unscientific cult and declaring it unethical for physicians to associate professionally with chiropractors. Such a strong statement was met with great resistance by chiropractors, who felt their opportunities to earn a living were being threatened.

In 1976, five chiropractors filed a lawsuit in federal court that the AMA, the American Osteopathic Association, the American Hospital Association, the American College of Radiology, the Joint Commission on Accreditation of Hospitals, and several other organizations and individuals had participated in an illegal boycott designed to destroy the chiropractic profession (*Wilk v. American Medical Association*, 735 F2d 217 7th Cir 1983). Several additional lawsuits were filed against the AMA and others in state courts and one suit was filed by the Attorney General of New York. The thrust of the argument was that since chiropractic was a licensed profession, any attempt to eliminate it was a violation of antitrust laws (Magner and Barrett, 1998).

The stakes of such an endeavor were high: if chiropractors lost their argument, they could be faced with substantial legal expenses. Additionally, if they lost, chiropractors had no other defense since they based the suit on a single legal argument. If they won, according to antitrust law, they would be entitled to triple the amount of damages and the AMA could end up having to pay the attorney's fees for the plaintiff, a sum expected to be in the millions of dollars. As a hedge to these risks, many plaintiffs negotiated and settled their cases in such a way that a favorable verdict would simply prohibit the AMA from being able to infringe upon physicians' rights to decide with whom they should maintain a professional relationship (Newborn, 2008; Long, 2013).

The *Wilk* case, named after one of the plaintiff chiropractors in the case, went to trial in 1980. After eight weeks of testimony, the jury found that the defendants, the AMA, were innocent. Upon appeal two years later, an appeals court overturned this verdict and ordered a new trial on the assertion that the original judge had misinterpreted the law. In essence the appeals court ruled that the issue was less about chiropractic and more about suppressing competition within medicine. The appeals court also contended that while the evidence showing "that chiropractic is in fact quackery," the amount of evidence presented by the AMA at the initial trial could have unfairly prejudiced the jury. To be fair, the amount of evidence presented by the AMA at this initial trial was indeed substantial—much of it came from documents obtained from chiropractic schools and internal documents from chiropractic organizations—and it showed a concerted effort to mislead the public and engage in dubious practices (Magner and Barrett, 1998).

Before the second trial, the remaining parties who had not already settled agreed to a bench trial (meaning no jury) and to waive their claim to damages. Chiropractors were content to have the case decided and hopefully, to have the AMA refrain from maligning their profession. In 1987, in a U.S. District Court in Chicago, Illinois, the judge ruled that the AMA had in fact violated the Sherman Antitrust Act. A federal appeals court upheld this decision and the U.S. Supreme Court declined to hear the case (Neborn, 2008).

In writing the opinion on the case, the District Court judge, Susan Gezendanner, pointed out that the AMA had acted improperly when it created the committee on quackery and engaged in a written and verbal campaign against chiropractors. The judge also ruled that the changes made by the AMA to their policies, where the AMA revised its declaration and said instead that physicians "shall be free to choose whom to serve, with whom to associated, and the environment in which to provide medical services," were insufficient, given the harm that had been inflicted on the chiropractic profession (*Wilk v. American Medical Association* 671 F. Supp. 1465, N. D. III. 1987; Magner and Barrett, 1998).

As some observers have noted, the concern by the AMA was not so much to destroy the chiropractic profession, but in using scientific methods for patient care. However, the court ruled that the manner in which the AMA went about voicing and applying its concerns did not need to be as damaging to the chiropractic profession. What is noteworthy is the following commentary from the judge's opinion in the case:

> None of the court's findings constituted a judicial endorsement of chiropractic. All of the parties in the case, including the plaintiffs, and the AMA, agreed that chiropractic treatment of diseases such as diabetes, high blood pressure, cancer, heart disease, and infectious disease is not proper and that the historic theory of chiropractic that there is a single cause and cure of disease was wrong. . . . There was evidence that the chiropractic theory of subluxations was unscientific, and evidence that some chiropractors engaged in unscientific practices. (*Wilk v. American Medical Association* 671 F. Supp. 1465, N. D. III. 1987; Magner and Barrett, 1998: 140)

The case was a clear victory for the chiropractic profession and put the medical profession on notice that they could not simply malign chiropractic medicine. Many chiropractors today refer to the case as a landmark moment in the history of the profession and its professional legitimacy (Newborn, 2008).

MEDICARE AND INSURANCE COVERAGE

According to some observers, as the result of a massive lobbying effort during the 1970s, chiropractic treatments were granted coverage under Medicare and Medicaid, along with worker's compensation and many commercial health insurance policies. The law took effect in 1973, and limited coverage to manual manipulation of the spine for "subluxations demonstrated by x-rays to exist" (Magner and Barrett, 1998: 128). One observer noted that the politics of the discussion resulted in members of Congress wanting Medicare to pay for something related to chiropractic care and accepted a loosely worded definition of subluxation for which payment could be made. It read: "an incomplete dislocation, off-centering fixation or abnormal spacing of the vertebrae . . . demonstrable . . . to individuals trained in the reading of x-rays" (Magner and Barrett, 1998: 128).

This decision was controversial from the beginning, but the upshot was that the rate of billing for chiropractic services skyrocketed. It also set off what has been identified within the profession as the "golden age" of chiropractic, since full reimbursement for treatment was usually approved. Given that the definition offered above was so ambiguous, it also led to a whole assortment of treatments being submitted by chiropractors, almost without any level of accountability (Simpson, 2012).

In 1986, the U.S. Department of Health and Human Services' Office of the Inspector General (OIG) reported that chiropractic treatments between 1975 and 1984 were among the top ten billed procedures under Medicare in 1983. The report also pointed out that the guidelines contained specific instructions of the types of conditions for which Medicare would reimburse chiropractors for treatments offered (Moran, 1986).

However, some critics have argued that this led chiropractors to "back door" billing (knowing what Medicare would not pay for led to chiropractors billing for subluxations that met the guidelines rather than for the actual treatment provided; see Moran, 1986). The concerns raised in the 1980s about questionable billing practices and outright fraud were reiterated in several reports by the OIG since the initial finding. In its most recent account on Medicare fraud and abuse, the OIG reported that there was approximately

$502 million paid to about 45,000 chiropractors for their services in 2013, but chiropractors also have the highest rates of improper payments from Medicare. Most of these improper payments were due to billing for maintenance therapy or other questionable treatments (Murrin, 2015).

DISCUSSION

As was mentioned, the use and popularity of alternative medicines today mimics the public's approach to it in the past. While many historical accounts have an overly critical tone when describing magnetic healing and other forms of alternative medicines, suggesting that the public was less educated about non-traditional forms of treatment, such practices are alive and well in contemporary America (Offit, 2013).

Even today we see an increasing mistrust of physicians and traditional medicine, not because of a lack of understanding of disease or because of the absence of scientific principles to explain various treatment modalities, but instead because the public believes physicians have been co-opted by pharmaceutical companies to promote and use a wide array of drugs to alleviate symptoms (Johnmar, 2015). In place of a mistrust based on competence, the American public appears to be increasingly turning to alternative remedies out of a fear that medications have too many side effects and the motives behind care by physicians are colored by financial incentives offered by these companies (Johnmar, 2015).

The need for additional drugs to counteract the side effects of the initial ones, which also produce side effects, leading to the need for additional drugs, has created a spiral of confusion and concern by patients and the public alike. Added to this dangerous treatment formula are the addictive properties of some drugs, such as opioids, the abuse of which, even those who hold a legal prescription for them, is now being heralded as an epidemic in this country (Center for Disease Control, 2017).

Thus, the mistrust by the public, along with the general dissatisfaction with traditional medicine, with many patients feeling as though their doctors and traditional medical providers lack compassion or concern for their well-being (Campbell, 2012), is a considerable and powerful influence on the public's desire to look for other means to solve their health issues.

However, these alternative medicines are not without their weaknesses. Similar to criticisms of chiropractors who blindly followed B. J. Palmer as he changed philosophies and techniques regularly, criticisms are being levied at the general public for its nearly fanatical fascination with all-natural products and alternative forms of medicine. Organic foods, New Age medicines, including energy work and supplements, are a multibillion dollar a year industry—with critics arguing that the public is just as immune from rational thought about their effectiveness today as they were about magnetic healing and elixirs and healing potions in the early nineteenth century. As the poet and philosopher George Santayana once said, "Those who cannot remember the past are condemned to repeat it" (Santayana, 2006).

Additionally, the issues surrounding the legitimization of chiropractic medicine through licensure and, more practically, through acceptance by insurance companies, have modern day significance. As we will see in subsequent chapters, what may be occurring is that chiropractic treatments, particularly their minimal impact on patient care, are a source of attention by insurance companies, who may see these treatments as more of a luxury item than a necessity. Such a narrowing view of chiropractic has resulted in many insurance companies eliminating or severely curtailing reimbursement for such treatments.

A potential unintended consequence of curtailing the use of chiropractic treatments as part of insurance coverage is a greater willingness by chiropractors to engage in questionable billing practices and even outright fraudulent ones. The issue of insurance coverage will be covered in the larger conversation about health care reform, but Medicare fraud is a salient issue both in terms of the economic costs and in efforts to legitimize the profession.

Finally, improvements in the quality and content of chiropractic education have potentially contributed to enhancing the credibility of the profession. Because the issue of training is critical to the future of the profession, particularly in light of the health care reforms occurring in the United States, an entire chapter will be devoted to this topic as well.

In the next chapter we offer insight into the nature of chiropractic medicine in South Carolina and introduce those participants in the study who played a key role in its overall success. While it is possible that the nature of chiropractic medicine may be different in this state than others, largely the result of the influence of two regional chiropractic colleges in the area, in many ways the issues in South Carolina are nearly identical to those included in national-level conversations about chiropractic medicine.

REFERENCES

American Medical Association, Department of Investigation. 1966. Educational Background of Chiropractic School Faculties." *Journal of the American Medical Association* 197: 999–1005.

Benedetti, Paul and MacPhail, Wayne. 2002. *Spin Doctors: The Chiropractic Industry Under Examination.* Toronto, ON: The Dundurn Group.

Campbell, D. 2012. "Doctors Accused of Lacking Compassion in Survey of Patients." *The Guardian,* September 27th. Available at https://www.theguardian.com/society/2012/sep/27/doctors-lacking-compassion-survey-of-patients

Center for Disease Control. 2017. *Opioid Epidemic*. Available at https://www.cdc.gov/drugoverdose/epidemic/index.htmlhttp://www.Civilwarhome.com/civilwarmedicine.htm

Flexnor, A. 1910. *Medical Education in the United States and Canada: A Report to the Carnegie Foundation for the Advancement of Teaching*. New York: Carnegie Mellon Foundation.

Foner, E. "Why Reconstruction Matters." *New York Time*s, March 28th. Available at https://www.nytimes.com/2015/03/29/opinion/Sunday/why-reconstruction-matters.html

Friebert, J., Wraight, J., Hagan, K. and Carter, H. 1994. *From Quackery to Bacteriology: The Emergence of Modern Medicine in the 19th Century*. Toledo, OH: University of Toledo Libraries.

Harrison, E. 1995. "A Brief History of D. D. Palmer," *The American Chiropractor*, January to February, 31–42. Available at http://www.vcu.edu/engweb/eng372/intro.htm

Homola, S. and Barrett, S. 1999. *Inside Chiropractic*. New York: Promethus Books.

Johnmar, F. 2015. "The Pharma-Physician Trust Gap that's Hiding in Plain Sight." *MediaPos*t. Available at https://www.mediapost.com/publications/article/263087/the-pharma-physician-trust-gap-thats-hiding-in-pl.html

Keating, Joseph. 1991. "Introducing the Neurocalometer: A View from the Fountain Head." *Journal of Canadian Chiropractic Association* 35(3): 177.

Keating, Joseph. 1993. "Old Dad Chiro Comes to Portland: Rediscovering DD in Oregon, 1908-10." *Chiropractic History* 13(2): 37.

Keating, Joseph. 1995. "Shhh! Radiophone Station WOC is on the Air: Chiropractic Broadcasting." *European Journal of Chiropractic* 43: 21–37.

King, L. S. 1982. "Medicine in the USA: Historical Vignettes: Medical Sects and their Influence." *Journal of the American Medical Association* 248: 1221–1224.

Long, P. H. 2013. *Chiropractic Abuse: An Insider's Lament*. New York: American Council on Science and Health.

Magner, G. and Barrett, S. 1998. *Chiropractic: The Victim's Perspective*. New York. Prometheus Books.

Mesmer, A. 1888. *Animal Magnetism*. New York: Appelton and Company.

Mills, C. W. 1959. *The Sociological Imagination*. New York: Oxford University Press.

Moran, W. 1986. *Inspection of Chiropractic Services Under Medicare*. Chicago, IL: United States Department of Health and Human Services, Office of Inspector General, Office of Analysis and Inspections.

Murrin, S. 2015. *CMS Should Use Targeted Tactics to Curb Questionable and Inappropriate Payments for Chiropractic Services*. Washington, DC: United States Department of Health and Human Services, Office of Inspector General. Available at http://www.chiromedicare.net/wp-content/uploads/2015/10/2015-OIG-Report-on-Chiropractic.pdf

Newborn, H. 2008. "The AMA Conspiracy to Contain and Eliminate the Practice of Chiropratic." *Natural News*, available at http://www.naturalnews.com/023857_chiropractic_AMA_the.html

Newborn, H. 2010. "How the Neurocalameter Changed Everything." *ChiroUnity*, available at http://chirounity.com/1090/how-the-neurocalometer-changed-everything

Offitt, P. 2013. "Alternative Medicines are Popular, but do they Really Work?" *The Washington Post,* November 11th. Available at https://www.washingtonpost.com/national/health-science/alternative-medicines-are-popular-but-do-any-of-them-really-work/2013/11/11/067f9272-004f-11e3-9711-3708310f6f4d_story.html?utm_term=.1a9e744f6407

Palmer, D. D. 1910. *The Chiropractor's Adjuster: Science and Art and Philosophy of Chiropractic.* Self published textbook.

Santayana, G. 2006. *The Life of Reason: Five Volumes in One*. New York: Echo Books.

Simpson, J. K. 2012. "The Five Eras of Chiropractic and the Future of Chiropractic as Seen Through the Eyes of a Participant Observer." *Chiropractic and Manual Therapies*, 20: 1.

"State by State: Comparing Chiropractic Scope of Practice." 2014. *Dynamic Chiropractic*, September 1. Available at http://www.dynamicchiropractic.com/mpacms/dc/article.php?id=57118

Wardell, W. 1992. *Chiropractic—History and Evolution of a New Profession.* St. Louis: Mosby.

Woodlief, A. 2012. *Introduction to American Romanticism.* Available at https://excellence-in-literature.com/introduction-to-american-romanticism-by-ann-woodlief

Chapter 3

The Chiropractic Experience, the Setting, and the Cast

Given that over half of the population in the United States has never been treated by a chiropractor, it is likely that little is generally known about what happens in a chiropractor's office or the types of treatments that occur there. There are over 200 different formally identified techniques used in chiropractic medicine and likely many others that have been developed by individual practitioners for their patients. In the initial portion of this chapter, we will focus attention on a user-friendly description of what happens when a patient comes to an office for treatment and a general description of some of the more popular techniques used by chiropractors.

This chapter will then offer insight into chiropractic medicine from the perspective of participants in the study in South Carolina, who were instrumental in providing background, insight, and referrals to other chiropractors in the state. This "snowball sampling" method is a common one used in ethnographic research. The profile of participants is offered not in an effort to generalize the findings to the larger population, but to understand the context and nuances of the subjects studied (Bailey, 1996). Such is the case here, where sociological studies of chiropractors have been absent in the literature for many years and none have explored providers in South Carolina.

THE SETTING OF A CHIROPRACTIC OFFICE

For those who have never been treated by a chiropractor, the experience could be an intimidating one. An initial trip to a chiropractor's office might be similar to going to the doctor or dentist. While not all doctor's offices are bad places to visit, there is often an atmosphere of what I call "clinicalness" to them; where the smell of disinfectant is present, the organization of the office is rather orderly and regimented, especially in a large practice.

Given that the nature of medicine has changed in recent times, where doctors now often have as little as ten minutes to spend with a patient, such volume often does not lend itself to a relaxed and casual atmosphere. In fact, one of the criticisms of traditional medicine has been that patients often feel that their providers are not attentive to their needs (Laidman, 2012). This is in addition to patients being forced to wait beyond their scheduled times in the waiting room to see their provider. At times, these delays can be quite long.

Perhaps it is intentional, then, that many chiropractic offices make a concerted effort to create a relaxed, casual, and welcoming atmosphere. Upon entry into many chiropractic offices, for example, one is immediately confronted with smells of scented candles or some form of aroma therapy that is soothing and relaxing. There are often very comfortable chairs in the waiting area and children's toys are typically present; in some cases an entire section of the waiting room is cordoned off as a miniature playground for young children. In addition, there is often bottled water, coffee, and other drinks and treats for patients as they wait to see the chiropractor. The décor of the waiting rooms tends to be contemporary, although some older chiropractic offices still have original or minimally upgraded features, where paneling or old carpet and art work are present. It is unclear whether this is a result of neglect, reluctance to upgrade due to costs, or an attempt to convey a more retro style in that particular office. In any event, the staff is almost always welcoming and friendly, and the receptionist usually knows a fair amount of personal information about each client.

It is quite common to hear a brief conversation between patient and staff concerning family, job situation, hobbies, or other things that are important to the patient. This familiarity might be intentional, where the staff keeps a cheat sheet about patients who have scheduled appointments or it may be that a closer relationship between patients and staff develops because they tend to visit the practice more frequently. Patients who have unscheduled visits, also known as "walk-ins," are also known to most of the staff. This may be due to the fact that they too visit the office more frequently because they have reoccurring injuries or engage in activities that aggravate conditions that require regular attention.

For whatever the reason, the atmosphere in all of the chiropractic offices I visited was upbeat, casual, and friendly, and the staff was a critical part of that process. As any medical provider who owns or operates a practice will confess, the front office is a central component of the success of that business. Employees who understand their role and are able to help patients solve their problems, whether it be due to billing, scheduling, or other challenges, not to mention those who embrace the idea of customer service, are integral to the practice. As many doctors have pointed out in my conversations with them, often they are unaware that a patient has left their practice because of being treated poorly by the staff until long after they are gone.

Whether it is because chiropractors are very mindful of the need for such staff and select employees with apt skills to deal with patients or because patients are only there a short time for each visit, this friendly and casual approach appears to be a noticeable theme in those practices that have a front office staff. Many chiropractors, particularly sole providers, attempt to reduce overhead costs by assuming the role of scheduler, billing person, compliance person, and other roles in addition to treating patients. This is likely the case in those practices that are small, have just begun operations, or where the provider is having difficulty meeting expenses. In those instances, the chiropractor serves several roles and it is important that he/she offers the same level of knowledge of the patient's personal life and willingness to assist them with billing and other problems during the visit.

In those chiropractic offices that diversify their treatments beyond chiropractic adjustments, there is a concerted effort to display the products sold or the services provided. For example, in one office where the chiropractor is very involved in providing and promoting nutritional supplements to patients, an entire wall displays an assortment of vitamins and other pills and creams. Those offices where the chiropractor offers weight loss programs, exercise gear, posters, weight scales, and motivational displays to encourage patients to maintain their efforts at losing weight are prominent. Most chiropractors have small sections of the waiting room (and some in treatment rooms) that display creams, equipment, and other items designed to serve as muscle relaxants, exercises, or other items designed to assist patients in maintaining their health.

Upon entry into one of these offices, the patient or visitor is greeted by a staff member, who is near the entrance and there is usually some type of check-in procedure to validate that they have met their appointment. Some of the more successful chiropractors use iPads as part of a system, where patients can check in and out, along with using that same tablet to pay their bill after their treatment. Some chiropractors have a staff person who serves as a receptionist to schedule appointments by phone or in person, as well as serving as the billing person for the practice. They are also the ones who handle the payment for services. This multifaceted role likely gives the staff more contact and interaction with the patient, and this likely results in learning more about them and their interests.

After the patient checks in, and, assuming they are not directly taken to the treatment area or room (some chiropractic offices are open spaces, with minimal barriers between the waiting and treatment areas), there is usually some sort of PowerPoint slide show on a large-screen television that offers motivational statements, medical information about the value of chiropractic treatments, or suggestions about some of the supplemental treatments available by the chiropractor. In some offices patients are introduced to new products being sold, such as lumbar support pillows, that are put in every chair in the waiting room, or floor mats that provide additional cushioning and support.

While all of these sources of stimuli are occurring, the chiropractor is seeing and treating patients and his/her voice can be heard counseling and educating them. At times the patient is asking questions about certain injuries or treatments while at other times, the chiropractor is recounting information about the value of chiropractic treatment and what it is doing to improve the patient's condition. Initially, I worried about such conversations within earshot of other patients and wondered about HIPPA violations, but after a time, it became evident to me that these were standard comments, almost script-like, that were told to all patients.

I also wondered if regular patients became accustomed to the monologue-like mantra and tuned the chiropractor out, unless he/she provided new information. At times, some chiropractors would point out a new study or a recent statistic about the number of people dying each year from medical malpractice, the number of people who sustained certain types of injuries, or a statistic about a recent health trend, such as the opioid epidemic. Whatever the topic, inevitably the conversation would result in some type of endorsement of chiropractic medicine and how the patient made the right choice in coming to see this particular provider.

The conversations with patients also typically involve comments about improvements that the chiropractor has seen in the patient, either in their range of motion, mobility, or in the chiropractor's clinical assessment of the movement of the joint or area of concern. In addition, the provider typically commented on how much better the patient is going to feel with additional treatment. In all the observations of interactions with patients, I never heard a chiropractor suggest that a patient was not improving or was not responding well to treatment. While all of what is presented to patients by chiropractors might be true from a medical perspective, some patients feel as if this is a form of salesmanship that makes them wonder about the effectiveness of chiropractic care. As one patient pointed out,

> I come in here and usually Dr. Mike does the same treatments on me, he does my back, my hips, and then my neck. And then I lay on another table and he does the same things he always does. This happens no matter what I tell him is wrong with me. If my middle back hurts, if my lower back hurts, it's always the same thing. Once in a while my elbow hurts and he adjusts that, but it's always

> the same treatment and it's always the same comments. "You're getting better, I can tell. Don't you feel less pain after a visit?" There are times when I wonder if the guy needs the validation that what he's doing is working because he's not sure that it does. But how can it be the same thing every single time? And I like the guy, don't get me wrong. He is very encouraging and always saying nice things about the things I'm doing in my job or my family. But it just makes me wonder if he says the same thing to every patient.

This patient's comments are similar to what others have offered to me in many other chiropractic offices. Some of it may be intentional, where the chiropractor has tried to use the power of suggestion with the patient to have them actually feeling better, and, to be fair, it is not unreasonable to ask a patient if they felt that a particular adjustment or treatment was effective. The difference appears to be in the motive behind the questioning. Does the patient feel that the chiropractor is trying to find the best treatment for his/her patient and wants feedback or is there some other motive, such as making sure the patient continues to return for additional treatment? Of course, we cannot know the actual motives and both may be operating at the same time. However, this portion of the typical interaction was noteworthy in my own observations of patients as well as in their independent accounts of what it is like to be a patient of a particular practice. These interactions have been studied elsewhere and while the focus was not so much on the patient's perceptions of the experience, the social interaction was part of an overall impression management characterized by Goffman's work (see Cowie and Roebuck, 1976; Goffman, 1969).

As was mentioned in the previous chapter, Cowie and Roebuck (1975) offered insight into the nature of social interaction within a chiropractic office. Serving as a member of the staff, Cowie, one of the coauthors of the study, was able to observe how and in what ways the front office learned about the patients' needs, interests, and issues, and then relayed them to the doctor prior to receiving their treatment. Drawing heavily on a Goffmanian framework, particularly as it relates to the notions of impression management and controlling the patient's understanding of the role of the chiropractor, this study offers great insight into how marketing efforts are supplemented by the staff, who encourage patients to refer their friends and relatives to the office for care.

By providing a safe and sympathetic atmosphere, one that is often at odds with the patient experience in traditional doctor's offices, Cowie and Roebuck (1975) concluded that there is an element of trust that is created between the patient and the provider. In addition, like the earlier studies, much of the impression management performed by the chiropractor is an effort to manage the stigma of being a member of a "tainted" profession.

Most of the treatments offered by the chiropractors lasted about five to ten minutes, depending on the patient and his/her condition. At times, additional treatments, such as traction, massage therapy, or trigger point therapy, were offered, but generally speaking, a patient's visit lasted less than fifteen minutes, including the time spent in the waiting area. As one chiropractor pointed out,

> See, most of my patients want to get in and get out. They want their treatment and want to be on their way. That's not how I like to practice. I prefer to spend time with them, get to know them and their lives, so that we develop a relationship that goes beyond the simple treating of their problems. But a lot of people are busy, they are doing lots of things and need to get this done so they can continue with their active lifestyle. So I try to meet them where they are and give them what they need. Sometimes patients only want to get treated and have their symptoms relieved. I tell them I can do that, but it won't help them in getting healthy. The reasons they have to keep coming back to me are what's causing them the problem, but a lot of patients only want to deal with the symptoms rather than the cure. So for these patients, I try to keep it simple and fast, but I always remind them that this is their choice and I'll help them anyway I can-but there's only so much I can do with what they've given me to work with.

Another provider offers this account:

> Listen, most people don't like going to the doctor, they don't like going to the dentist and the last thing they want to do is spend a lot of time sitting around waiting to get what they need. So I try to move them in and out as fast as I can. That helps them, given that it's what they want, and it helps me, so I can treat more patients in a day. I would like to give them more, but especially with younger people, like the college kids I tend to see, that's all they want. Adjust me and get me back on the field or doing what I want to do. That's it.

I had the opportunity to talk to a few patients about their experiences with the practice and the process while they were waiting to be seen by their particular chiropractor. In describing the process, one patient said,

> I like the fact that I can go whenever I want, get treated and be on my way. I don't have time to sit around a doctor's office for an hour and a half waiting for an appointment that starts an hour later than I was scheduled. Even then, I get into the treatment room and it's another fifteen or twenty minutes of waiting. With Dr. Dave, I go in, I don't wait that long, and I get treated. It doesn't take but five or ten minutes and I'm out the door.

Another patient says they like the regularity of treatment:

> I think going to the chiropractor is a lot like brushing your teeth. . . . You need to do it regularly even though you know eventually you're going to have to see the dentist about something more serious. Dr. Smith told me that if I came regularly, I wouldn't have the problems I was experiencing, and he's right. I come about once every two or three weeks, even if I'm not feeling any pain, and he makes sure I'm all set regarding my back issues. The fact that my insurance doesn't cover it means I have to come out of pocket for the treatments, but it's worth it. If I throw my back out and am on the couch for a week, how much is that costing me?

One of the more skeptical and cynical patients offered this commentary, where he equated the chiropractor with a car salesman, particularly as it related to developing a long-term relationship.

> I have been giving a lot of thought to whether this is really worth it for me. I know they all talk about wanting a long-term relationship instead of my coming just when I need treatment, but why would I show up if I'm not in pain? When the staff and Dr. Mike talk about a relationship, it feels a little like a car sales pitch—they don't want to sell me just one car, they want me coming there for every car I ever buy. But I don't go to the dealership for maintenance, it's too expensive and they rake you. I think they should just let me come when I need it and not make me feel guilty about not coming once a week or whatever. This isn't the way to build a relationship, it's a way to make people feel like they are getting scammed.

Most of the patients generally believed that their chiropractor was trustworthy and kind, and really wanted to help them. They offered comments where the chiropractor was able to remember something they had told him/her either in a previous visit or some time ago. Most said that their primary care provider could not do that, unless it was in the chart. Many patients also commented on the fact that they had seen other chiropractors in the past and they had a bad experience, meaning the adjustments made the injury worse or simply did not help. These patients typically then point out that once they started seeing their present chiropractor, things improved dramatically. This indictment of chiropractors based on one experience is a common theme. As one chiropractor astutely pointed out,

> When I meet someone and they tell me they had a bad experience with a chiropractor and that's why they don't want to see another one, I often get frustrated by that. I mean, I never touched you or put my hands on you, so why would you think that what that last guy did would be what would occur if I treated you? I mean, you go to a restaurant and have a bad meal, you maybe have a problem with that restaurant right? You might give them another chance, but more than likely you won't go back there. But do you avoid all restaurants because you had

a bad experience with one of them? But that's how people see chiropractors. . . . It's like if one guy does something wrong, we are all bad. So when I hear people say, "well, Dr. Steve, I wasn't going to come and see you because I had a bad experience with a chiropractor, but my friend told me to give you a try, but I was skeptical," it really makes me wonder what patients think of us. Have they ever had a bad experience with a physician and did that keep them from seeing a different doctor? It's crazy.

POPULAR TECHNIQUES AND TREATMENTS

While there are a host of techniques and treatments used by chiropractors, in part depending on the nature of the injury or illness the patient is experiencing, and in part based on the particular philosophy of the provider, there are a number of techniques that are used by most chiropractors on patients. While some can be quite technical in their description, what is offered here is a more streamlined and simple explanation of what happens when a patient is treated by a chiropractor (Painter, 2011; see also Bergmann and Peterson, 2010).

Diversified Technique—Perhaps the most common procedure used by chiropractors is called diversified. This manipulation/adjustment involves a quick thrust that often results in the popping noise that many patients are familiar with in chiropractic. While the popping noise is not part of the adjustment, rather it is the release of a buildup of the gases in the joint, the thrust is an effort to realign the spine to its proper form.

Extremity Manipulation—A variation of a diversified technique involves applying the adjustment to areas other than the spine, such as the elbow, shoulder, finger, ankle, and so on. These types of adjustments are said to improve the range of motion of the joint and relieve pain from problems such as carpel tunnel syndrome, tendonitis, and other issues.

Activator Method—This instrument is sometimes used instead of manual manipulation by using a small device that delivers a more superficial thrust to perform the adjustment. It is used for some patients who want a gentle adjustment or in places where a hand-borne manipulation is not possible.

Gonstead Technique—This technique, although still performed by hand, differs from the Diversified technique because it focuses on a certain type of joint manipulation. Gonstead is said to be a rather specific adjustment that more precisely focuses on the affected area, rather than the entire spine.

Cox Flexion/Distraction—This technique is used to treat cervical and spinal disorders or injuries and to increase mobility in the spinal joints. A special table is used where the spine is elongated and bent forward. In other words, this technique is similar in many ways to a form of traction, where the spine is stretched to release tension in the spine or neck region.

Thompson Technique—This technique is a variation of the Diversified that uses what is known as a "drop table." Essentially, portions of the table can be moved up in small increments (often fractions of an inch) to provide a fulcrum from which the adjustment is applied. When the chiropractor performs the thrust as part of the adjustment, the section of the table "drops." The purpose of this is to open or free the joint during the adjustment. The drop also assists in the thrust, meaning it requires less physical effort by the chiropractor.

Sacro-Occipital Technique (SOT)—This technique uses a triangle-shaped blocks placed under the pelvis as the patient lies on their stomachs. This is designed to treat lower back problems. In addition, slow pressure on the problem area can be used, but the idea is that providing the patient with a flat and balanced surface can relieve some of the muscle spasm and pain. At times the wedge-shaped blocks are all that the patient needs to reduce the spasm and pain.

Applied Kinesiology—This approach to chiropractic care measures skin temperature and muscle strength in a particular area to identify an injury. The rationale is that muscle areas that are weak in strength are said to be identifiable by certain physical tests, and where those muscles are weak, trouble spots of illness or disease can be seen. While not exactly a test of raw strength, applied kinesiology carries with it a great deal of controversy and a lack of scientific proof despite the fact that about a third of all chiropractors use it (Russell and Rovere, 2009).

NIMMO/Receptor Tonus—This technique is based on the idea that muscular spasms can influence joint functioning. As muscles go into spasm, they may limit the range of motion of a joint. By applying pressure to the muscles in spasm, often called trigger points, the muscles relax and return to their normal functioning. When that occurs, the bones and joints begin to move normally as well.

Palmer Upper Cervical/Toggle Recoil—This technique is a generic term to describe the range of techniques used to adjust areas of the neck. Some techniques focus on the upper cervical area. The belief is that treating these areas addresses problems throughout the body. Sometimes chiropractors will refer to this as adjusting one's Atlas or C1 to refer to the first cervical vertebrae.

Logan Basic—This technique involves the chiropractor using a light pressure, usually one finger, applied to the ligaments in the patient's sacrum. Correspondingly, a similarly light pressure is applied to the areas that are in spasm or painful. This gentle technique provides the opportunity for the muscles to return to their normal length and functioning (Painter, 2011).

In addition to these specific techniques there are a range of treatments that fall under the general heading of Cranial Technique which focus on adjustments to joints of the skull, similar to SOT for the spine. Also, as was mentioned in the use of the activator, there are a range of treatments where the provider will use adjusting instruments to apply a more accurate adjustment where a very specific and precise manipulation is needed (Painter, 2011).

In a 2000 study by the National Board of Chiropractic Examiners, entitled *Job Analysis of Chiropractic*, efforts were made to find some of the most common techniques used by providers. As was mentioned, while there are nearly 200 identified techniques used in chiropractic medicine, and, undoubtedly variations of these techniques used by individual practitioners, the analysis reveals the most common techniques practiced by chiropractors (Painter, 2000).

As Table 3.1 shows, a vast majority of chiropractors use a diversified technique on patients and most do some form of extremity adjustment. The latter is particularly noteworthy for chiropractors who specialize in sports injuries. The other techniques are used in varying degrees by chiropractors, but this may also be a result of the training they received in their chiropractic college. Logan University's Basic technique, for instance, is an important part of that program, while other chiropractic colleges may not offer it at all or only as an elective course. Other chiropractors may use activators when the patient is uncomfortable with the sounds generated from an adjustment or have difficulty with the physical positioning needed to perform a particular technique. Some chiropractors use the activator method, for example, when a more forceful thrust is not required. Thus, the percentages of use may not be based on popularity or effectiveness alone. Rather there may be other reasons why a particular provider uses one technique over another. Of course, the

Table 3.1 Most Frequently Used Techniques by Chiropractors

Technique/Procedure	*Frequency of Use by Chiropractors (%)*
Diversified	95.9
Extremity manipulating/adjusting	95.5
Activator Methods	62.8
Gonstead	58.5
Cox Flexion/Distraction	58.0
Thompson Technique	55.9
Sacro-Occipital Technique (SOT)	41.3
Applied Kinesiology	43.2
NIMMO/Receptor Tonus	40.0
Cranial	37.3
Adjustment Instruments	34.5
Palmer Upper Cervical	28.8
Logan Basic	28.7

Source: Painter, 2011.

patient's needs and injuries largely determine the course of treatment, but these are the most common techniques a patient might see when visiting a chiropractor for treatment.

SOUTH CAROLINA AND ITS CHIROPRACTORS

In many ways, South Carolina as a state tends to have a personality that is similar to many chiropractors—independent, strong-willed, and determined to do things in its own way. South Carolina became the eighth state to ratify the U.S. Constitution in 1788 and the first state to vote to secede from the Union in 1860. The state's residents have a number of strong positions on social issues, such as same-sex marriage, unionized labor, evangelical religious beliefs, and gun control. South Carolina is named in honor of King Charles I of England, under whose reign the English colony was first formed, with *Carolus* being Latin for "Charles" (South Carolina State Library, n.d.).

According to the U.S. Census, in 2015, South Carolina has approximately 4.9 million people, about a 6 percent increase since the Census in 2010 (U.S. Census, 2014). South Carolina is the twenty-third most populous state in the country, and comprises forty-six counties. Its capital is Columbia with a population of about 135,000 and the largest city is Charleston, though it is only slightly larger than Columbia. The Greenville-Anderson-Mauldin area is the largest metropolitan area with nearly a million people living there (South Carolina State Library, n.d.)

As of the 2015 census estimate, almost 77 percent of the population are white, about 13 percent black or African American, 14 percent were of Hispanic or Latino origin, and about 5 percent were Asian, with about 1 percent American Indian and Alaska Native; a small fraction, less than 1 percent, were Native Hawaiian and other Pacific Islander (U. S. Census, 2015).

Many large corporations have moved their locations to South Carolina. Boeing opened an aircraft manufacturing facility in Charleston in 2011. In 1994, BMW launched a production facility in Spartanburg County, while many other corporations are moving factories and headquarters to the state as well. There is also a strong military presence in the state, particularly in Charleston, with several military contractors located in the region.

South Carolina is said to be one of the most politically conservative states in the country and this is reflected in its laws regarding issues related to gun control and public opinion about topics such as abortion and same-sex marriages. With regard to gun control, a recent article pointed out that South Carolina is part of a growing trend in this country regarding people's need to protect themselves. According to a recent Pew Research Center poll, 57 percent of respondents felt that gun ownership protects people from crime and

52 percent felt that it was more important to protect the right of Americans to own guns than control gun ownership. In South Carolina, a state dominated by conservative politicians, 80 percent of Republicans felt the same way as the Pew respondents about gun ownership. Not surprisingly, gun laws in South Carolina are generous to gun owners (Smith, 2015).

As it relates to same-sex marriage, a recent study by Winthrop University found that 52 percent of South Carolina residents still oppose gay marriages. This differs significantly from polls conducted in 2011, where nearly 70 percent of residents opposed it (Newsmax, 2013). Some might see this as a promising trend; however, national opinion polls show that over 55 percent of the public supports same-sex marriage.

Thus, it is fair to say that Conservative views on a variety of issues dominate South Carolina and this is often revealed in the state's laws regulating certain types of activities. However, the history of the state indicates that it is steadfast in its belief in autonomy, in independence, and in embracing the notion of state's rights to regulate life in the state.

South Carolina Chiropractors

In South Carolina, as in many states, licensure of chiropractors is perhaps the only meaningful way of exerting any significant form of social control over the profession. Without a license to practice, chiropractors run the risk of criminal and civil penalties. The South Carolina Department of Labor, Licensing and Regulation, the Division of Professional and Occupational Licensing (LLR), is the government agency responsible for collecting, disseminating, and maintaining information about chiropractic licenses. Unfortunately, this agency does not keep extensive records on licensure for chiropractors. This makes it virtually impossible to determine the total number of chiropractors, largely due to the fact that the LLR collects data for a two-year period and then erases it.

What we do know is that there has been a significant decline in the number of chiropractors who did not renew their licenses between 2016 and 2017. In fact, according to that agency's account, there was a 38.6 percent decrease in the number of chiropractors who did not renew their licenses, from 1,753 in November 2016 to 1,098 in February 2017. Such a dramatic decrease would normally be a cause for concern. I contacted the LLR office to learn more about how the information is collected and maintained. I explained my initial finding and asked for another account of the records in March 2017.

A reexamination showed the new number to be 1,144. While improved, the number still represents a significant decline, 34.7 percent. I wondered if the data provided was an aberration, so I asked for five-year's worth of data to see if the trend had been a consistent one. This was when I learned that the agency only keeps records for two years. When I asked the LLR staff about a possible explanation for the significant decline, representatives from that agency pointed out that the decrease in licensure renewal meant the licensee either moved out of the area or chose to close their business. Such an alarming trend is noteworthy but not inconsistent with what some chiropractors have offered in their own assessment of the profession. As Jim, a chiropractor in the study, pointed out,

> I know a lot of guys who have simply gotten out of the profession all together because they can't make any money. The insurance reimbursement, along with the fears about a Medicare audit, have caused some guys to simply do something else. I mean some of the old timers might have gotten out because of all the new requirements and how the insurance companies are making it too much of a hassle. If these guys were older and had made their money, maybe they sold their practice but my guess is that a lot of them, and a lot of the newer guys just walked away from it.

Any profession that witnesses a nearly 40 percent decline in its members should be a significant cause for concern, even if there were too many providers in the marketplace. Several attempts were made to contact the South Carolina Chiropractic Association, with the goal of making them aware of the problem as well as to gain some insight as to why these developments have occurred. Unfortunately, after repeated efforts to schedule an interview, there was no response from representatives of the organization. This is a bit of a curious finding, but as Jim points out, it is not unreasonable to conclude that many have left the profession due to the inability to generate sufficient revenue.

Alternatively, this dramatic decrease in the number of chiropractors who renewed their licenses may be a result of attrition as many older chiropractors simply retire and no longer practice. It is also possible that the nature of the profession, where, depending on the types of techniques used, is physically demanding. Chronic injuries as a result of performing chiropractic treatments usually result in a shortened career or a diversification of the practice. As one elderly chiropractor points out,

> You don't see too many 58-year-old chiropractors like me. The body tends to break down long before that. So what guys tend to do is either hire associates to come in and do the heavy lifting, while they continue to promote the practice, or they sell their practices outright and retire. This is less likely these days because it takes so long to build a practice and sustain it that guys aren't likely to just walk away or sell it. Another option would be for guys to change the configuration of their practice, where they don't do as much chiropractic adjusting, but maybe they do more weight loss or nutrition supplements, or that kind

> of thing. Many older chiropractors also start using the Activator, which is a tool that allows for adjusting the spine, but is much less taxing on them. It is a less forceful adjustment, but it prolongs their careers . . . and it gets patients back in the office more frequently as well.

One provider pointed out his experiences with the South Carolina Chiropractic Association. He says,

> I tried to become involved in the state organization for chiropractors. What a waste of time. They don't do anything and when they have meetings, either by district or collectively, they only talk about the same things—and it becomes more of a support group discussion—"Hey, how do you generate new patients? How do you bill for this particular thing? How many times have you advertised here?" The organization doesn't seem all that interested in doing anything meaningful. Maybe they do but they aren't really communicating it to the members. So I think guys just stop participating. Maybe they are more involved with the state legislature and getting things passed but I haven't seen anything from them in a long time. So why would anyone spend the time and money to be a member if they don't get anything out of it?

While many state professional organizations do not have an active membership, where many professionals prefer to affiliate more closely with their national or regional associations, there may be a number of similar problems with the South Carolina Chiropractic Association as well. However, one has to wonder if the organization is remaining up to date on current issues within the profession. A review of their website, for example, shows that they are using figures and statistics from 2004. This may be a minor oversight, but coupled with the lack of response about a potentially serious issue in the profession, along with comments by providers about the value of the organization, one wonders if its role within the profession is highly valued.

A Profile of Chiropractors and Chiropractic

While there were forty chiropractors formally interviewed for this study, there is some commonality in terms of the characteristics of this cast. This is not to say that all chiropractors are the same, but the following descriptions characterize some of the more common features of the chiropractors interviewed. This selection offers a profile of participants based on factors such as age, length of time in the profession, philosophy of treatment, and other characteristics to provide a general understanding of the entire group. This study included chiropractors across South Carolina, but clustered in the largest area of the state. In reviewing the demographic figures about participants in this study, a number of trends were identified.

For instance, a vast majority of chiropractors involved in the study were male, white, married, and trained either at Life University or the Sherman College of Chiropractic. This makes sense, as was mentioned, given that these chiropractic colleges are in close proximity to the state; one is located in Marietta, Georgia, while the other is located in Spartanburg, South Carolina. The influence of these two colleges likely results in self-selection for this particular study. Given the strong philosophical influence—both schools believe in the concept of vertebrae subluxations and are more likely to reflect "straight" chiropractic ideas.

Most of the chiropractors in the study were married, many with children, and have been practicing in the state for ten years or more. This means many came into the profession prior to Obamacare and have experienced the significant changes health care reform has had on the profession. While this was not a topic directly explored during the interviews, judging from the conversations it appears that a vast majority of chiropractors in the study profess some type of Christian belief system. Table 3.2 offers a brief summary of these demographic variables.

As Table 3.3 shows, in assessing the nature of their particular practice, if they owned one, this group of participants were typically solo practitioners. This is still very common in the profession, where large groups, such as those found in traditional medicine, are rare in chiropractic medicine. This may relate to the greater need for autonomy and independence of chiropractors, as mentioned in the opening chapter.

The use of associates remains a common theme in the profession. However, there are many issues that arise from such an arrangement. For instance,

Table 3.2 Demographic Information on South Carolina Chiropractors

Variable	*Percent/Frequency*
Gender	
Male	88% (35)
Female	12% (5)
Race/Ethnicity	
White	98% (39)
African American	2% (1)
Asian	—
Hispanic/Latino	—
Other	
Age (years)	
26–35	10% (4)
36–45	65% (26)
46–54	15% (6)
55–64	10% (4)
65 and older	—
Total:	40

Table 3.3 Distribution of Type of Practice by Gender

	Type of Practice		
	Solo	*Partnership*	*Associate*
Male	30	2	3
Female	3	2	0
Total:	33	4	3

for a new or recent graduate of a chiropractic college, who may not have the financial resources or patient list to sustain a practice, working for an existing provider is a way to develop their craft as a chiropractor as well as to learn more about what it takes to operate and sustain a practice. While there are many models to choose from in terms of compensation, often the chiropractor will hire an associate at a base salary with a series of incentive bonuses if the associate reaches certain performance benchmarks. This is not uncommon in medicine, and there are some arrangements where an associate can "buy into" a practice and eventually purchase it outright from the owner. Unlike traditional medicine, however, where physicians' starting salaries, depending on the specialty, range from $200,000 to $600,000 (Miller, 2016), the starting salaries for chiropractic associates can be rather low, often as little as $35,000 to $40,000 per year. Yet the cost of attending a chiropractic college can be as much as that of attending a medical school.

As many chiropractors have noted, the associate experience can be a difficult one, particularly since many recent graduates have significant student debt. As one participant in the study noted, there is another dimension to chiropractic as it relates to the treatment of associates that is less than flattering. He says,

> If you asked ten chiropractors, about eight of them will know and understand this phrase. It's "chiropractors eat their young." Ask around and see how many understand what this means . . . most do. So you get a chiropractor who graduates fresh, and they take them on in their practice as an associate. What does that mean? It means they're 1099, it means they don't pay them anything, they send them out to these spine screenings to drum up business. And as these chiropractors start bringing in three or five new patients a week and they start building the practice and they get a hundred patients, the chiropractor says to the associate, I don't think I need you anymore. . . . So then he sends an email to all his patients and says, well, doctor so and so has left the practice but I'm happy to continue to take care of you . . . and that's how they build their practice . . . it's pretty ruthless.

Just about every chiropractor I spent time with who has been in the field has offered an account of this experience. While they may reflect on what happened to them retrospectively as a positive event later in their careers, almost all talk about how they were exploited by a senior colleague early in their careers. Joe had this to say:

> There's all kinds of formulas, but chiropractors are notoriously cheap and the biggest complaint I always here is that I felt like I was slave labor. And I had that experience too. I got out of school and had a guaranteed salary of 200 dollars per week. Moved to Michigan from SC. So I was making less money than I was making in chiropractic college waiting tables. But I had a good bonus system because the guy was the VP of the state chiropractic association and he travelled a lot. But after working for him for a year, and building his practice . . . I built his practice. I had more people seeing me than were seeing him, he basically came in and said "Well we are going to rework things." I worked Tuesday Thursdays and Saturdays and he worked Monday Wednesday and Fridays. And I covered for him when he traveled. He said "What we're going to do now is, just going to have you work every day for the same amount." So when he traveled I earned the same amount. . . . I didn't get a hundred dollars covering for him when he was gone. So I went from making maybe six or seven hundred dollars a week sometimes to maybe three hundred a week if I made my performance bonus or whatever. So, I was slave labor and I was really treated very poorly even after I had built his practice and done well. But the bottom line is this: I got my hands on more bodies than I ever would on my own. My first week in practice I probably adjusted two hundred patients, where if I started out I'd have been lucky to see two patients. So I sat at lunch time and learned the billing, learned how to do scheduling, learned how to do x-ray reports, learned how to manage patients, how to table talk and do all these things. So even though I had a crappy experience it was invaluable in what I learned. I think that's one of the things that young guys don't get now, even if you were slave labor, you probably were making as much or more than you've made probably at any other time in your life, and you probably had the opportunity to learn a lot. . . . Did you learn a lot? Or did you just go in everyday and come in as late as you can and leave as early as you can?

Doug, another chiropractor who has been in the profession for over a decade, offers this account of his experiences, which is what led him to leave his initial practice as an associate. He says,

> When I first graduated from chiropractic school, I went to work for this guy in Louisiana. I was all excited to start my career and thought this would be a cool place to begin. Well, this was a large practice and this guy was really about the money aspect of chiropractic, not the treating patients part. The first day I get there he sits me down and gives me all these scripts that he wants me to memorize on how to convince patients to purchase these maintenance plans, either weekly or monthly. It was crazy, all he wanted me to do was build his practice for him and he saw that as my primary function. I didn't want to tell patients to buy things

> they didn't need and it was a really hard time for me. I felt in the interview like he was going to be a good guy to work for and that I would be able to take care of a lot of people, but he was just a businessman. I was trying to figure out how to get out of my contract when Hurricane Katrina hit and wiped out the entire area. So what does this guy do? He fired everybody in the office so he didn't have to pay their payroll tax or any of the other things. Then he basically tried to hire them back once everybody was allowed to come back into the area. So I was lucky to get out of that and then I came to South Carolina and opened up a practice with a friend. He moved to Michigan after a while and I bought him out, so here I am now. But in the beginning, I couldn't believe how poorly that guy in Louisiana treated me and his staff. But I have heard lots of stories from other chiropractors over the years about their experiences right out of school or when someone needed to work as an associate in addition to owning their practice.

Joe, who had a negative experience initially as an associate years ago when he graduated from chiropractic school, is now in a position to hire other associates. As he describes, his experiences with them have not been positive, but he attributes it to a generational phenomenon, where chiropractic graduates' expectations are too high. He says,

> I have had associates before. And this one guy in particular, he wasn't interested in doing much to learn about the business or about how to run a practice. He came in twenty minutes late and wanted to leave as early as he could. He said, "I'm not getting paid enough to be committed." That sounds a lot like Millennial generation sense of entitlement. I hired Michael to work with me until I opened my other practice. And what I did was I put him out there, Mondays Wednesdays and Fridays and I went out there Tuesdays and Thursdays and he covered for me here on those days.
>
> So we flip flopped back and forth. And he had a good salary and a good bonus incentive. And he was making pretty good money . . . and it was getting better all the time. The problem was he just wanted to show up at 8 o'clock in the morning and leave at six o'clock at night and didn't want to invest time in building that practice. He didn't want to be there after work, going to the Lions Club, didn't want to be there before work going to the café downtown where all the city leaders are . . . and I needed someone who was going to be out there, wanting to be a leader in the community. So after a year, I looked at Michael and said, you're not going to be the doctor out here anymore. You've done good, but I need someone who wants to be out here and wants to commit to that community.
>
> I need someone who wants to live out here, raise a family out here, and be a community leader. That's not you. You don't want to live out here. You want to hang out, drink beer on weekends and chase girls and I understand that. You're a young guy, you're just out of school. But that's not what that practice needs. We need to commit to that community. He looked at me and said you're right. So I said you've got two options, you can shake my hand and say goodbye, or

> tell me to screw off and say goodbye, or you can come back and work with me full-time in the other practice, but I'm going to hire a full-time doctor at the other office . . . if you still think you have something to learn.
>
> So he said he wanted to come back here and work with me. . . . So he came back here and I hired another doctor to work there. That guy I hired at the other practice lived in the town where the office was located, his wife grew up there, he wants to be there so he's perfect for the practice, so I just sold the practice to him after two years. And that was sooner than I had planned on. . . . I was going to give him an option to buy into the practice at like 25 percent and eventually buy in at 50 percent, but I just decided that I wanted to go ahead and give him the opportunity to buy the whole practice, because I knew he wanted it and financially I wondered if he was going to be able to do it. So we worked it out so he could, and gave him an opportunity to get his own practice. . . . It was good for him, it was good for me. . . . But I haven't had a lot of good experiences with associates.

While there are many models on how to operate a practice, with some having administrative staff while others do not, or where the types of ancillary staff (such as acupuncturists or physical therapists) present varies quite a bit, most of the chiropractors who owned or operated practices made use of massage therapists. Interestingly, few chiropractors employed massage therapists directly. Rather, a common practice was to rent space to an independent massage therapist (or in some cases an acupuncturist) and allow that provider to operate a separate business from within the practice.

Such an arrangement is mutually beneficial for both parties and relieves the chiropractor of any tax obligations or other obstacles related to hiring and employing massage therapists. In most cases it is described as a "straight up" business arrangement, where the massage therapist has complete control over his/her own schedule, handles their own payments to clients, and maintains responsibility for their own separate business. It is likely that such an arrangement emerged as a more common one after insurance coverage changed so that massage therapy is no longer covered under most insurance plans. Thus, there is no financial incentive for chiropractors to have massage therapists on staff, particularly if patients do not seek out massage therapy in addition to chiropractic treatment.

THE CAST

Dr. Doug is around thirty-eight years old and has been in practice for about twelve years. He operates a solo practice in town and has supplemented his practice with a weight loss program. Doug grew up in the upstate New York area and has many friends and associates who are chiropractors. He is single and lives alone, but has a wide circle of friends. Doug's practice is, as he puts it, mildly successful, although as he points out, Obamacare has placed a major obstacle in the way of his success. He says:

> When my partner and I started this practice, it was before Obamacare, but after the golden age of chiropractic. That's when you got reimbursed for everything you billed for. Then it was a little harder later on, but still manageable. But when Obamacare hit, like the first two years, man, I was really worried about whether this was going to work or not. I mean, for me, the problem isn't as bad. I'm not married, I don't have kids, I'm still a younger guy, but for some of the other guys in practice, it was probably a pretty big shock. I know I will be all right if things get skinny for a while, because I don't have a lot of expenses, but I did worry about my student loan debt.
>
> That's a lot of money—it's like owning a house. For a while I had to let my payments go because we weren't making a lot of money in the practice, especially when the economy tanked. . . . NOBODY was coming in for treatment. I tried to negotiate my payments but they weren't interested in working with me. So I had to default for a few months. But then I started this weight loss program and things have improved. I'm not really in a location where we get a lot of walk in traffic, so I have to make sure patients schedule appointments because it takes a bit of energy and time to come to this office.
>
> But I probably should be doing more in terms of screenings and clinics and advertising too, but I'll tell you, it is just exhausting. You have to come to the office, treat patients all day, keep up with the insane medical notes they now ask you to keep on every patient, so that by the time I'm finished for the day, the last thing I want to do is grab some stuff and go talk to people and convince them to come to my practice. And then you get there and other chiropractors are already there—and you worry about poaching existing patients from other chiropractors. I should be doing more, I know that, but it just doesn't seem to happen with all the other demands placed on me.
>
> And it's just me. I don't have a partner so anything that has to happen has to be done by me. I've been doing this for more than twelve years now and I'll tell you, I don't know how these other guys do it. I wonder how many are still in the business. It has gotten so hard to earn a living like this. And I won't do these practice building seminars, they are so . . . I mean, ethically, I just can't get behind misleading patients just so I can earn a living. I have to have some type of integrity for myself and those guys are all about the money.
>
> I didn't get into this business to make a lot of money, I did it because I wanted to help people become healthy. But that's not what it is any more for me. . . . It's just work. The weight loss stuff has helped because you can see tangible results as people get healthier, but I worry about the profession and about whether or not I'll be doing this in another ten years.

Doug is a Sherman graduate and says he decided to stay in South Carolina after graduation because the weather there was better than in the Northeast and because he had made lots of friends while in chiropractic college. Being a former athlete, his active lifestyle, and an assortment of injuries originally attracted him to chiropractic medicine. He says,

> I never really wanted to go to medical school, not that I could get in anyway, but I went to a chiropractor after getting hurt and he was able to help in a way that my regular doctor could not. So it became an area of interest for me. I looked around at all the chiropractic colleges in the country, even the one in my home state, but it was hard to figure out all the differences. Sherman seemed to make the most sense at the time, but looking back, I'm not sure I was adequately prepared when I graduated. I'm not even sure I believe in the idea of the subluxation anymore either.

Dr. Joe is an older chiropractor, who has been in practice for nearly forty years. A Sherman graduate, he says he started out believing in the philosophies of Sherman, but in developing his practice he has introduced some level of diversification, largely the result of nutritional supplements. A visit to his office shows a wall-length display of vitamins and other nutritional supplements that he uses in his practice.

Joe has been rather successful in his practice over the years, in part likely because he was able to experience that golden age of chiropractic, where many providers earned high salaries as a result of generous reimbursements by insurance companies. Joe has a thriving practice, seeing upwards of 250 patients per week, even though he is the sole provider in the office, many of whom are regular patients, who come in for adjustments and to purchase dietary supplements. Joe has opened other practices in the region and has made use of associates in the past, but currently is trying to develop a retirement plan to exit the profession. As he points out,

> There aren't many 58-year-old chiropractors who are still working in the office like I do. It takes its toll on you and I have to maintain a strict diet and fitness regime in order to be able to treat as many patients as I do. But I'm starting to wear down, I can feel it. I've been doing this a long time and I've had some success, largely because I believe in educating my patients to take responsibility for themselves.
>
> I call myself a wellness doctor, because chiropractic is only one part, an important part, but only one part of what I do. My goal is to get people to understand what they need to do to get and stay healthy. And because they are active and are moving, they are going to need my help in a variety of ways. Some will only come in when they are injured or in pain, which is fine, but I try to get them to see the value in a health regime that will keep them from getting injured as often or to minimize its effect when they do. It's a lot easier to get someone moving again if that joint isn't fired up because they have been coming to see me regularly than if they waited and now it's not moving like it should be.

A visit to Joe's office demonstrates both his commitment to helping his patients and the success of his practice. There is a steady flow of patients in the waiting area and Joe does a good job of minimizing the time they have to wait to be seen. Some of these patients have scheduled appointments, but many are walk-ins. Joe handles all of them with efficiency and grace. His treatment area is open so that patients can hear him talking about a variety of topics to the person lying on the treatment table.

At times there is repetition to the mantra, almost as if he's reciting from a script, but the patients do not seem to mind. He says that the repetition is good because it reminds them of the need to make the changes necessary to maintain their health. As he begins to talk about what he does as a wellness doctor, he points out that getting healthy is not simply a matter of periodic monitoring. Rather it involves regular visits and with it come regular educational opportunities. He says,

> But if you come once a month, we can maintain the work that we've done. Just like, you lost all that weight, you can't go back to eating the way you did before. You don't have to be on negative calorie intake because you're trying to lose, you're able to loosen up your diet a little bit, but you still need to eat right to maintain. Same thing for exercise. You got in shape so you can run the Cooper River Bridge. Now if you run twice a week, next year you don't have to train for the Cooper River Bridge. But if you stop running all together, you got to start all over and you have to start training about twelve weeks out to get ready for that bridge run. So maintenance is not new to chiropractic, it's been around forever. So that's what I try to help my patients understand. I want you to feel better. And you're gonna start to feel better after about four or five adjustments. But here's why you don't want to quit. Because symptoms are always the last thing to show up in a health condition, and they're the first thing to go away. That's the way the body's created.
>
> The body will shift and rotate, the body will compensate, it will do everything it can to keep you functioning normally, because that's how we're designed. But finally, it gets so bad where the check engine light comes on or the oil light comes on. Now you got two choices. Stop the car and put some oil in it and solve the problem, or you can reach up under the dash and pull that wire out that makes the light go off. So that's what I try to help people understand.
>
> The symptoms are going to go away pretty quickly, but it's going to take some time to make the problem go away that we saw on the x-ray, that degenerative disk or that bone spurring. We've got to get that joint healthy again. That takes about 60–90 days, now the great thing about that is once we do that, you don't have to go back and do it again, but it takes some time to do that initially. Once we do it, then it is all about taking care of it and maintaining it. So I give my patients those options, I say, if you want to use chiropractic as like a pain pill or muscle relaxant for temporary pain relief, you can do that and I'm happy to help you with that. Just understand that this is what you're doing and over time this problem will progress and get worse.

> If you want to correct it, we can do that too, you have the choice, here's the information, you make an informed decision. So that's what I give my patients, I give them information and a lot of it. . . . Sometimes people go, "there goes doc again" [smiles]. It's not unusual, and I'm not bragging or anything, and my staff will attest to this, she has heard multiple patients over the years say I learn more when I come into this office than I have any other place I've ever gone. I learn something new every time I come into this office. And that's the type of atmosphere we try to create.

Dr. Jack is a chiropractor in his early forties and has a thriving practice in the downtown area. Recently he has expanded his operations beyond one office to include two others, where he has hired young associates to run those practices with his guidance. Jack is very friendly and quick witted and has a knack for observing subtle cues about people and integrates them into his conversations with people and his patients. Married, with two young boys, Jack is a former athlete who has an acute business sense. His relationship with his patients is very informal, he does not wear a lab coat, and his tie, coupled with his sneakers, sends an interesting message about how serious he takes himself, but recognizes the importance of looking professional. As he tells the story,

> I remember when I was first starting out, when we moved here in 2002, I met this real estate guy . . . this bigger than life Southern guy. He liked me so he pulls me aside and says (in this deliberate Southern accent), "Son, there's only two things you need to remember to be successful in business. One, always be honest with people. You never know who is related to somebody around here and if you don't treat 'em right, it will bite you in the butt. And two, always wear a tie. You can be the biggest dope on the planet, but if you wear a tie, people will think you are at least making an effort to look professional" [laughs]. I still remember that guy and I think of him every morning when I put on my tie. Now I might wear running shoes 'cause I'm on my feet all day and the pants I wear might not be expensive because I'm getting up and down on my knees treating people, but I always wear a tie. It was good advice because even now I look like I'm thirteen years old, so patients want to feel like they can trust that I know what I'm doing, but I have never forgotten that.

His demeanor is self-effacing and the conversations with patients often resembles guys meeting at a restaurant or ball game—they cover a lot of topics and Jack brings up details of previous conversations or his recollections of the patients hobbies' or interests. This comes remarkably, despite the fact that he says he often will not see a patient for months at a time. Unlike Joe, who professes the need to see patients on a regular basis, Jack takes a different approach, encouraging patients to only come see him when they need it.

These differing points of view will be the topic of the next chapter, but one gets the distinct impression that Jack is the kind of guy people like to be around, they often leave his office giggling at a one liner he's offered, often at his own expense, or something that is going on in the world that he connects to their lives.

Jack's practice is a thriving one, with upwards of 300 patients a week. But he maintains a conservative décor in the office and he does not have treatment rooms. Instead, he has a treatment table in his office, where patients come in and chat and then receive an adjustment or other treatment. The office is adorned with crayon drawings from children, likely his own or those of his patients, and while he has multiple framed certifications hanging on the walls, ostensibly to document his competency for new patients, many of these frames have sketches of various types, clearly created by children, taped to them. So there is a bit of incongruence to Jack, one that I think he enjoys presenting to people. But this laid back attitude and less conspicuous presentation of self hides a very thoughtful and shrewd understanding of his profession and of issues related to it.

In an effort to diversify the practice, Jack leases out space to an acupuncturist and to a massage therapist, to provide the kind of comprehensive treatment that patients want or need. However, he is quick to point out:

> The acupuncturist or the massage therapist, they don't work for me, I don't work for them. If you want the services they provide, you work through them. I don't get a kickback from their operation and I don't try to refer people to them either. I let them know it is available, but that's it. I believe in letting the patient decide for themselves and they know I'm not pushing them one way or the other. That's why I'm successful. People trust me and know that I'm not looking to make a buck from them. It's also why I don't charge nearly as much as other chiropractors. So they know, I can go to Jack, he knows what he is doing, I only need to go to him when I need to, and he's less expensive than everyone else. I don't need to make $2,500 out of every patient. I can make $200 or $300 from them and not see them for a year. But I also know they'll come back because they feel better and I'm honest with them.

Our conversations typically focused on the health care reform efforts going on, or, what he calls the "big play" in medicine, which involves taking the general practitioner out of the equation and allowing the patient to have more autonomy and control over the type of treatments he/she receives and how they are delivered. Jack's observations will be a critical part of the discussion on health care in Chapter 7.

Dr. Kat is one of the few female chiropractors who participated in this study. She graduated from the University of Western States Chiropractic College about three years ago, and is still relatively new to the profession. She works as an associate for multiple chiropractors, giving her a perspective on the profession that is rather different than her more senior colleagues like Joe. She has also moonlighted as a bartender in an effort to offset the salary she receives from these other opportunities. Kat grew up in South Carolina and her father is a primary care physician. She says,

> I had a general biology degree but most people I went to school with, there were a couple that had either kind of like, degrees in literature or something like that. . . . And you can, technically, just get a certain number of prerequisites and go straight into chiropractic school as long as you have those. Technically you can do that for medical school too, but the competitiveness is, just no way. In chiropractic school you can do that, so there were like two or three people that were like 20 years old who just knew what they wanted to do in high school. And they did what they did to get into chiropractic school.
>
> [So are you from the Portland area?]
>
> No, I grew up in South Carolina and went to USC for my undergraduate degree. And then actually worked at MUSC for about three years, because I was kind of thinking after I got out of school that I wanted to get my Ph.D. So I was working in a cancer lab, working with chemo prevention with natural options. But I liked my side of it, but when I looked at the other side of it, like what the PI of the lab had to do, with the stuff that you're actually doing when you're making a living, I just. I wasn't into it. Living on soft money is hard.
>
> [So what led you to chiropractic?]
>
> My dad is a family practice physician, and so I had . . . I just grew up seeing his hours . . . and he's not even a specialist, just basic family practice . . . and he's still . . . you miss a lot of stuff, because you're taking care of your patients . . . lot of holidays he had to work on and recitals and I was just like, that's not for me. I mean it is a good paycheck, but there's always a sacrifice to be made, and I mean, especially now, I remember when I was younger and he had his own smaller practice, it was before EMR, it was not nearly as bad when he was a junior associate. I mean, oh my gosh, I rarely go home, and he's almost 70 years old and I rarely go home and he's not sitting there entering charts on his computer, at home, on his time. I have it here, but it isn't anything like that. . . . I mean, our coding is so minimal.
>
> [So how did you pick the school in Portland?]
>
> So I did some research and I knew I wanted to leave the state for sure. I just wanted to see some other places, but when I was doing research, that program in particular has a lot of emphasis on evidenced based practice and so to me, like I feel there are different kinds of chiropractors and there are those who are focused on the innate flow and all this kind of stuff. And for me, I need something a little more medical than that. So that program was just a better fit for me.
>
> [How has it been since you graduated?]
>
> My first job was in Denver. It was high volume, and I got really good, I had to, I was seeing like 40 patients a day. I probably saw more people there than most people see their entire career in a conventional practice. And then I

> decided to move to South Carolina, I really took for granted what it was like to work for her, because I couldn't find anything that I felt comfortable doing. . . . And I have like three skills, I can do stuff in medical research, I can do this, and I can bartend. . . . I've got what it takes to survive and got all these other skills to get by. . . . I mean I was bartending for a while and making more money than I am now, honestly, but some people don't have those skills. . . . Like those people that go straight in . . . . They don't have any other skill set to tie them over until they can get their practice running. . . . And I just don't know how they do it.
>
> In my case, I'm okay with not starting out on my own . . . the deal I have here is perfect for me, it's a 60-40 split and I've been amazed at how many people have come in after only two weeks. But while the percentage isn't even, I don't have any of the overhead, the marketing, equipment, none of that. I just have to increase the volume, which I can do . . . and the chiropractor I work for has been telling people to come here because he has a lot of connections and patients that live in town, so he tells them to come here instead. I can make up the difference between what I need and what I make. I know everyone in town in terms of food and bev . . . . It's nice to have a side hustle you can rely on. So I guess I've had a really interesting time sort of navigating post-school employment.

As a relatively recent graduate, Kat has some insight into the chiropractic college experience and some of the challenges that graduates face regarding significant debt for attending. This relates to issues stemming from the costs of starting a practice as well as the reimbursement issues that characterize current insurance plans. Her insights and comments will be helpful in understanding the role that chiropractic colleges play in the profession in Chapter 6.

Like Kat, Dr. Kathleen is a relatively recent graduate, but unlike her colleague, Kathleen did not grow up in South Carolina and was trained at a different chiropractic college, National University. Kathleen is also a licensed acupuncturist and works as an associate for a chiropractor in an integrated medical office, with nurse practitioners and physicians on staff. The chiropractor leases space from the medical clinic and often collaborates with the medical team as the need arises. Her experiences are a bit different as a result, but several issues are of particular importance to her. She offers this account of how she got into the profession:

> I didn't want to go to medical school, I didn't try to get into medical school, I didn't want to do the pharmacology route. I think medicine has turned into a drug dispensary. I think true osteopaths, that's kind of the perfect mix of both. . . . I kind of wish chiropractic would go more in that direction instead of getting into the (whistles) stuff. Waving crystals . . . I wish we'd be more evidence-based, and if the profession would get on the same page we might be able to require that . . . the Board to do more studies to prove that it works.

I mean physical therapists do a lot of the same stuff that we do . . . and MDs have no problem referring you to a physical therapist in part because the physical therapists are all on the same page. Their education is very regulated, they all learn the same basic principles while they are in school.

I think chiropractic also attracts a certain personality type, a bit rebellious. . . . They like to be their own man, like to do their own thing, like to come up with their own ideas. A lot of them base their results on case studies in their own office . . . which could just be placebo. . . . I mean 50% of medicine is placebo . . . surgery, not acute stuff, but a lot of orthopedic surgeries have a lot of placebos, and pharmaceuticals . . . which is why a lot of drug companies . . . I mean it works for some people and does nothing for others. Along with your biochemistry too. I found chiropractic school to be very confusing [laughs].

[So why go?]

I didn't think it was confusing until I got about halfway through and then I was like, what the . . . This one guy is telling me one thing, this other guy is telling me something else. And then I'm going to this weekend seminar and they're telling me something else, and I'm like is it A, B, or C? laughs. And I'm more left brained, so I'm more comfortable with knowing this is what we're supposed to be doing versus, I get the art of it too, and the technique, where everyone has their own technique, but I like to know more about why what I'm doing is working . . . and they don't have that.

[It's interesting . . . so now three years out . . . what does it look like for you?]

I love working for the doctor who owns the practice. I kind of am on my own, and I'm still associated with him. So it's kind of a partnership, which is perfect for me, I can practice the way I want to, which is different from the way others wanted it. I worked for a couple of other chiropractors that wanted me to do the way they were doing it. And they wanted me to build their practice for them without much in the way of sharing the profits. So I think some guys take advantage of associates because they know they are at a disadvantage. And a lot of chiropractors do some creative billing. The first practice I worked for did a lot of creative billing and I turned them in and they ended up getting shut down. And the second guy I worked for was doing the same thing but he was so well established that they just didn't do anything about it.

What I like about this gig is that I can practice the way I want to and as long as I'm generating revenue for the practice and getting new patients, and I'm at least somewhat in alignment with what the guy who owns the practice wants, he's okay with me doing it my way. I can't afford to start my own practice and if this continues, I may not want to. But there are a lot of guys out there who are doing some crazy stuff.

When I got here, I grew up in Illinois, I met these chiropractors who were trained at Life or at Sherman and they were talking about all kinds of crazy pseudo-science and it sounded like religious fundamentalism to me. I had never seen any of that stuff at National and so I was like . . . ooookkkkaaaayyy. And got away from those guys. I think they don't do the profession a bit of good and keep us from getting the kind of credibility we need to have in order to continue in the future.

THE UNIQUENESS OF A PRACTICE

These five providers represent the range and scope of the group that participated in the study. A vast majority of chiropractors were men, with approximately ten to fifteen years of experience in the field. Most were trained either at Life University or at the Sherman College of Chiropractic. The difference, however, is that many proclaimed to be traditional chiropractors, who believed in the idea of the vertebrae subluxation, but many of their practices contained a variety of diversified items, such as nutritional supplements, weight loss programs, acupuncturists, and other alternative medicine treatments, including energy work and meditation. This would normally qualify the group as "mixers" but most claimed to want to retain the "basics" of "true" chiropractic treatments or made mention of the fact that they were a bit different. This belief in uniqueness of practice was a theme that ran through all of the interviews.

In fact, virtually every chiropractor interviewed made some sort of claim that their practice was very different and unique from others in the area. As Jack pointed out:

> My practice isn't like any of the other ones you'll see around here. I have a unique clientele, where my patients have median incomes of $200,000 or more. They are educated, smart, and are very active. I have people that fly here in their own jets to come see me for treatment. Why? Because they know what they are getting when they come here, they trust me, and they know I'm not trying to take advantage of them. Some of these people I only see once or twice a year, or when they need me because they've been injured. I don't ask people to see me for maintenance therapy. I let them dictate that—they know when they need an adjustment and then they come. I use an aggressive form of therapy that gets them back on their feet right away and don't charge them too much for each visit.

Another chiropractor, Dr. Ed, says his practice is different because he specializes in a particular technique called Active Release Therapy (ART). Essentially, ART is a treatment that focuses on adhesions or scar tissues in muscles. Essentially what happens is when a person is injured, muscle tissue is damaged. In response, the body replaces the damaged or injured tissue with scar tissue, sometimes called adhesions, that attaches to existing healthy tissue. Over time, however, these adhesions can grow larger and result in shorter and weaker muscles, which impact the person's range of motion and can press on nerves causing pain. ART uses hand pressure and stretching motions to eliminate these adhesions and release trapped blood vessels, thereby eliminating pain and weakness in the tissue. Many argue that this treatment is superior to traditional chiropractic and has demonstrated its effectiveness empirically. Ed's practice specializes in ART. He says,

> Well, what I use is what I call soft tissue work. Basically it is called ART or active release therapy. . . . Even now with people being more knowledgeable about their health, it is going to be patient education, but also too, it's that, I think we do a good job of keeping what we do a secret. I don't do any advertising. . . . But when we do it, do they know what you do in your office? A culture of humility. Like mine, okay, so we're going to do marketing, they need patients, but our marketing is going to be if you have back pain, come see us. If you've been in a car accident, come see us. But in our practice, we're going to be doing the ART and combined it with the adjustment. My two docs were at the home and garden show . . . had a booth there . . . doing ART screening . . . and people are like I didn't know chiropractors did this . . . this isn't chiropractic as I understood it . . . so things like that. Then the other stuff, you can't get everyone on the same page, but you have to stay true to your heart and at the same time, you have this number you're trying to reach. . . . So there's no quick answer, for me, what can we do currently? We'll educate people about it. . . . But it's not the whole infomercial stuff, too good to be true . . . because people won't believe you.

Still others focus on what they call rehabilitative work, which, from the descriptions offered, sounds a lot like physical therapy. As Josh describes, it is the kind of work used on patients with chronic injuries that seems related to chiropractic but really falls more in line with conventional physical therapy treatments. As Mike points out, making it as a chiropractor these days is difficult and, at times, one has to balance the ideology of chiropractic with the practical realities of other forms of treatment. He says,

> Okay so I do a lot of corrective rehab. Say someone has a flat cervical curve. I'll do a certain number of visits to get the joints moving, then I'll work on reconstructive therapies to start bringing the curve back. Like a posture pump, posture walk, and a series of things and then I check the x-ray in like three months and do my measurements. And when you see you it starting to come back, then I know we're on to something. And so does the patient. After 22 years it's nice to see that the principles still work, but the patients feel better, they see it. And then their health is starting to improve. We really express our lives through our nervous system.
>
> I've done . . . I'm 30 hours away from getting my diplomat, but I lose interest because I want to stick with the core. I used to do what's called Spinal Decompression. Goes totally against the philosophy of chiropractic but the way I got around it was that with me is who am I sending my bad disc patients? So this was my last ditch effort before surgery and 9 out of 10 times they got fixed. So to me that's still a win. But sometimes I have to get out of my own way with the philosophy thing, and I know that sometimes I think it has held me back but I want to be known as the guy who went down swinging and he went down believing.

Finally, one particular technique that appears to appeal to some providers is called the Blair technique. As Connie points out,

> The Blair technique does away with all of the cracking and noises of an adjustment and is much more specific. In a minute I'll show you the specific ways I mark the x-rays and the standard ones are and the ones I take in addition to that. But basically, it was developed, because Dr. Blair, who developed it in the 1950s, I would say, he was unhappy with the system of evaluating the upper cervical because the brain stem you've got your brain and your brain stem with turns into the spinal cord, so the most delicate part of your nervous system is in the top part of your neck, which is the smallest part of your neck. And there's 24 cranial nerves, off of there, so these green nerves are just some of the cranial nerves. . . . so you have cranial nerves 1–10, so I have a patient coming in right now who has bells palsey so I have numerous patients that helped, crazy enough, with heart problems because I took pressure off their vegal nerve.
>
> But what I find is, that when I take these precise measurements and x-rays and I do the precise adjustments, it affects a lot of different things in the body. And then my adjustments can actually be more gentle. But the biggest thing for me is that I have a bulging disk in my lower back and my left hip was always two degrees higher than the other. One of the reasons I explored this technique is because I would be in class and they would evaluate my hips and find like that my right hip was up. Then I'd get up and walk to the next class and get evaluated and they'd say the same thing.
>
> And I'm like something is causing this not to stay in alignment. And I hear this from patients too, they say, "well I get adjusted and I feel better but then it feels like it pulls back out again." And so the big nerves that control along the spine, the prime mover muscled, they are controlled by the upper cervical. And the trap muscles, and leviator muscles are controlled by C1. So when you address that, then people's hips level out and patients with problems like scoliosis is life changing for them. People feel the difference . . . and they can feel the difference when their neck is in or out of alignment, especially that initial adjustment is really profound. So I wouldn't do any other type of technique.

Some chiropractors attempt to focus on patients with unique needs, such as pregnant women. As Keith points out, he feels this puts him in a different category than what most chiropractors do:

> And honestly I don't know a lot of the other chiropractors so I tend to think mine is a small practice, but there are some that are high volume practices, where people are coming through . . . and I don't like that myself, so I have a pretty good relationship with my patients, and my patients keep coming back because they know me and trust me. And I wouldn't want to do this if I couldn't have that type of relationship. . . . and with a high volume practice would I be able to do that? I mean a lot of times, I get patients because they've been to high

volume practices. . . . This guy sees me for thirty seconds when I'm there, so they come to me.

So a lot of times I have patients that come in and say you charge more than this guy does, but usually they stick around because I try to offer a good quality service, but as far as challenges, it is just being able to afford someone at the front desk and to have the practice run more efficiently. I get a little bogged down with filing forms and returning phone calls. . . . I hate missing phone calls, but I don't want to leave my patients to answer the phone so, I'll call back and a lot of time people are Googling and they are going down the list and the first person who answers the phone, they go to them. So I realize we lose patients that way.

Parents always care deeply about their children's health and there's no time in a women's life that she's concerned about her health than when she's pregnant. And families who come in together for wellness care, they're coming in because they value the service, not because they have a back ache, once every four or five months. So I appreciate that they appreciate the care they receive from me. It's nice to be able to have a conversation about health when patients come in and not . . . and we have a lot of patients who come in and say I have back pain right here, fix it right here . . . um but those patients aren't going to be as happy in my practice as those patients who are coming in for the long haul.

Primarily we have a practice of OBs who send patients our way, if they've seen their patients. I've had patients who have been put on bed rest, 25 weeks, so they have another 15–17 weeks of pregnancy left. . . . where they were going to be lying in bed . . . for things like pubic dysfunction or something like that . . . and we can keep them walking throughout the rest of their pregnancy. Which makes the patient happy, they are able to keep working . . . and the OB isn't losing anything in terms of an office visit because they couldn't do anything anyway. So there's no loss for them. It's something where they say I have no idea what to do, and we do the same thing for them that we do for every other patient, so it's not like there's some magic formula for pubic dysfunction or sciatic pain, or whatever it is.

And I can never say I specialize in OB, it's prenatal care, and all the technicalities involved. They ask do you do the technique that turns babies. There's a technique specific for pregnancy called Webster technique and it deals a lot with the ligaments surrounding the belly and the uterus and the pelvic balance and that sort of thing. And almost without fail, I should be keeping track of the numbers, but almost without fail if the pelvis is in good alignment and the surrounding ligaments and fascia are right, the baby is going to come out head down. So we get a lot of referrals at 37 or 38 weeks, because they're telling the patient, go and try anything you want to try because it looks like we're going to have to do a c section if the baby. . . . So a lot of moms are saying, well, I don't want a c section, so I'll give it a shot. It's much better if they are coming in earlier than that, but that they're coming and OBs are willing to say try anything, kind of a left handed compliment, but they're willing to acknowledge that they're not the end all be all to the woman's medical care, which is healthy.

Thus, whether it was the clientele, where some claimed that their patients were from a higher socioeconomic bracket, or that their specialty of focus made them unique, where some catered to pregnant women while others focused on those with particular injuries or used unusual techniques, such as the Blair technique or ART, all claimed to be different from the norm. When I asked each of them about other chiropractors in the area, most could name one or two others, often former partners or associates with whom they worked or chiropractors who helped them get started when they arrived in the area. However, none had a real sense of the marketplace or the other providers in it. Perhaps this is why they felt their particular practice was so unique.

In sum, the observations and comments offered in this chapter provide a greater level of understanding of the dynamics of the chiropractic experience. By learning a bit about the techniques used, what it might be like to visit a chiropractor's office and/or receive treatment, along with a bit of understanding of the role of providers, such as how they organize their practice and whether they make use of other providers, we gain a glimpse of the micro-level interactions that take place in the profession. What follows are more macro-level descriptions of some of the key issues within the profession, including the perceptions of chiropractors themselves, and issues relating to what they think their role in medicine should be, the political and social divisions within the profession. These and other topics will be explored in the next chapter.

REFERENCES

Bailey, C. 2011. *A Guide to Field Research.* Thousand Oaks, CA: Sage.

Bergmann, T. and Peterson, D. 2010. *Chiropractic Techniques.* 3rd edition. New York: Mosby.

Laidman, J. 2012. "Patient Dissatisfaction Increases with Delays and Short Visits." *Medscape Medical News,* February 13th. Available at http://www.medscape.com/viewarticle/758566

Miller, P. 2016. "Survey: Starting Salaries for Physicians Skyrocketing." *AMN Healthcare*, June 9th. Available at http://amnhealthcare.investorroom.com/2016-06-09-Survey-Starting-Salaries-For-Physicians-Spiking

Painter, F. 2000; 2011. *Chiropractic Techniques.* Available at http://www.chiro.org/LINKS/ABSTRACTS/Chiropractic_Techniques.shtml

Russel, J. and Rovere, A. (eds.). 2009. "Applied Kinesiology." American Cancer Society *Complete Guide to Complementary and Alternative Cancer Therapies* (2nd ed.). American Cancer Society, pp. 160–164.

Smith, J. 2015. "SC Gun Laws: How they Compare Nationally." March 30th, *Newsmax,* available at http://www.newsmax.com/FastFeatures/SC-gun-control-gun-rights/2015/03/31/id/635249/

United States Census. 2014. *Table 1 Annual Estimate of the Resident Life Population for the United States, Regions, States and Puerto Rico April 1, 2010 to July 1, 2014.* Available at https://www.census.gov/popest/data/state/totals/2014/tables/NST-EST2014-01.csv

United States Census. 2015. *South Carolina Quick Facts*. Available at https://www.census.gov/quickfacts/

"Winthrop Poll: Most Still Oppose Gay Marriage in SC," June 4th 2013. *Newsmax*, available at http://www.newsmax.com/Politics/gay-marriage-poll-south-carolina/2013/11/04/id/534689.

Chapter 4

Scope of Practice

Mc: Talk to me about your ideas about scope of practice for chiropractors.
Jack: Well, that's a loaded question.
Mc: Why?
Jack: Well, because it's not so easy to answer and this is where people start attacking chiropractors.
Mc: Attacking them? Why?
Jack: Because they use this as a platform to criticize what chiropractic does and why we shouldn't be allowed to practice.
Mc: Does everyone who asks about your scope of practice do this?
Jack: Yes.
Mc: How then do you ever have an opportunity to talk about what you think what chiropractors should be doing if everyone in the profession thinks this is some sort of assault?
Jack: Well, we don't. I think chiropractors should define for themselves what their scope of practice is.
Mc: So no standards at all? Everyone gets to decide for themselves what they want to do with no accountability?
Jack: Right. I get to practice the way I want to without someone telling me what I can do or not do.
*Mc:*What about those guys you mentioned earlier who are bad for the profession?
Jack: Well, I don't like what those guys do, I think it's bad for the profession. And I won't do those things, but I don't want to tell them how to practice and I surely don't want someone telling me how to practice.

In the initial chapter, we examined how the public perceives chiropractors, including those who have been treated by chiropractors, as well as how the medical community has generally responded to the chiropractic profession and its providers. In the last chapter, we focused on a microlevel analysis of chiropractors and the profession: what do chiropractic offices look like and smell like, the sounds associated with a viable practice, and the interactional rituals that occur between patients and staff as well as between patients and the chiropractor.

We also explored how associates to a chiropractic office are used in the profession and some of the dynamics and challenges found there. At this point in telling the larger story of chiropractors, the reader should have some sense of what it is like to seek and receive treatment and have developed some understanding of the social relationships found in chiropractic medicine.

In this chapter we extend that understanding of the profession a bit further by examining how chiropractors see themselves: to the medical profession, to the public, to other alternative medicine providers, and, perhaps most importantly, how they see each other. This is important because, as we will see, the lack of internal consistency has plagued the profession's ability to organize itself as well as inhibiting its ability to gain credibility and legitimacy.

This discussion begins with an understanding of what chiropractors think their scope of practice should be—as we see in this opening vignette, the topic is a sensitive one for chiropractors, who often feel a sense of persecution and any questions about this issue, even innocuous ones, can evoke a defensive response. Throughout the study, when this subject came up, Jack's reaction was similar to those of many of his colleagues. Even when the question was rephrased by asking about a provider's philosophy of treatment, suggesting that their training guided how they currently practice, the question was often avoided or changed. It took quite an effort to reframe the discussion and return to the topic later but eventually most providers opened up about where they stood on certain issues like this one. Perhaps it was an opportunity to vent a little, or maybe the chiropractors saw that I was simply trying to understand the complexity of the issue, but it was quite a challenge throughout the study.

A key component to uncovering a particular provider's scope of practice seems to be related to the controversy surrounding the vertebral subluxation. Those chiropractors who truly believe in what we will call *sublux theory* tend to follow a certain philosophy of treatment about what they do, and, more generally, how all chiropractors should practice. Most chiropractors seem to be aware of their colleagues' different methods of treatment, and while they may criticize them for several reasons, they are quick to defend other chiropractors, even in the face of overwhelming evidence that their actions are questionable or even outright fraudulent.

It is also true that many chiropractors who subscribe to the belief in sublux theory have strong opinions about what the scope of practice should be as well as holding rather conservative views on topics related to the profession, such as whether or not chiropractors should be authorized to write prescriptions. Maintenance therapy is another topic of discussion that evokes strong reactions among chiropractors, particularly if it is considered a necessary component of a patient's treatment plan. Where one stands on any or all of these issues lends insight into the particular chiropractor's philosophy of treatment, and, by extension, their scope of practice.

Scope of practice is one of the most controversial issues explored in this study and the accounts offered by providers, coupled with an objective assessment based on the available literature, provide a rather fascinating and comprehensive exposure to chiropractic medicine. In addition, commentary from deans and provosts of many chiropractic colleges around the country are included in the discussion, most of whom are or were practicing chiropractors at some point in their careers.

Where applicable, accounts from physicians as well as comparisons to traditional medicine are also included to provide some balance about what chiropractors offer in their practices. Both chiropractic and traditional medicine contain a degree of inexactness about what is known about the treatments offered. In other words, some of the criticisms of chiropractic medicine might be warranted, but they must also be understood in reference to some of the same types of challenges seen in traditional medicine. While traditional medicine may have evolved further and more completely than chiropractic, largely due to its willingness to embrace its own limited understanding of certain diseases and illnesses, and while there have been some remarkable discoveries about a variety of treatments and illnesses, it is far from complete or perfect.

As researchers in the field of epidemiology have pointed out for years, there are a host of social, economic, and political factors that contribute to disease and illness. In addition, the role of the patient should not be overlooked in understanding their health and wellness—where their willingness to make lifestyle changes (or even to consistently take the medicine provided to them by doctors) also has a role to play in understanding health.

Thus, there are a multitude of factors that contribute to a person's health and realistically, all medical providers are limited to some extent with regard to what they can do to help patients get better. In the end, regardless of the treatments available or their overall actual effectiveness, it is the patient who has to decide what they want, what they need, and what they are willing to do regarding their own health. This is true for conventional medicine as well as for any advice or suggestions offered by chiropractors.

All that said, there is a significant amount of controversy and a good deal of internal strife within chiropractic medicine. Much of this has to do with the inability or unwillingness to adequately regulate members of the profession. The reason may be due to a fear of the loss of autonomy, as Steven points outs in the opening vignette, but some of it also relates to scope of practice and a lack of consensus on the boundaries of what chiropractors should be doing when they treat patients. These and other topics will be explored at length but the first, and perhaps most controversial, issue to address is the scientific validity surrounding the subluxation.

DOES IT EXIST? VERTEBRAL SUBLUXATION

At the heart of the discussion about the overall validity of chiropractic medicine in general and the scope of practice for chiropractors in particular is the debate about whether or not vertebral subluxations exist. If vertebral subluxations do exist, are chiropractors the most qualified to treat them and is that treatment more effective than other remedies, including allowing the injury to heal on its own without any treatment at all?

Recall that in chapter 2, the vertebral subluxation is often described as a condition caused by misaligned vertebrae in the spine impinging on the nerves surrounding them, causing pain and a lack of mobility in the joint. Proponents of the subluxation theory contend that impacted nerves can also interfere with internal organs, thereby causing disease. Realigning the vertebrae through manual adjustment, sometimes also called *spinal manipulation*, restores the spine to its proper configuration, thereby allowing nerves to function properly.

Critics of chiropractic medicine argue that vertebral subluxations do not exist and have never existed, and chiropractors are unwilling to admit that because it is what distinguishes chiropractic medicine from any other form of treatment. In other words, without the vertebral subluxation, the profession has no identity, credibility, or viability. While there are a host of books written that criticize the profession as either dangerous, quackery, or a form of con artistry, virtually all consider this topic to be a pivot point of legitimacy for the profession.

For example, in *Spin Doctors: The Chiropractic Industry Under Examination*, Benedetti and MacPhail (2002) point to problems with the existence of the vertebral subluxation from the early days of the profession. They argue that D. D. Palmer made up the existence of the subluxation and since then chiropractors have staked their professional identities on it. As they state,

> What chiropractors have been doing for the last century is trying desperately to show *how* Palmer's subluxation could work, rather than investigating *whether* it exists. Of late, chiropractic leaders have been boasting of the profession's evidence-based direction and its commitment to research. But little, if any, of that research is directed at the key question for chiropractic. (p. 59)

The authors go on to point out that the profession was created based on an undocumented assumption and yet its members continue to promote it as if it were real. Benedetti and MacPhail (2002) point to evidence to show that the subluxation is not possible scientifically and that even chiropractors have difficulty in identifying them. Many chiropractors today still claim to be able to identify and treat subluxations, but studies show that chiropractors have not been able to demonstrate this ability with any level of consistency or accuracy. In fact, some studies have shown that chiropractors often have difficulty definitively identifying a subluxation on an x-ray or accurately pointing them out in examining the x-rays of the same patient (Feise, 2001). Benedetti and McPhail (2002) use this as evidence to show that perhaps the reason for the disagreements or inability to identify subluxations is because they do not really exist in the first place. Benedetti and MacPhail (2002) argue the following:

> When B. J. Palmer taught chiropractic adjustments, he argued that the misaligned vertebrae above and below the spinal nerves could pinch them. However, as the science and anatomy behind it shows, vertebrae almost never pinch nerves and pinched nerves don't cause disease. Despite that, many chiropractors still offer it as an explanation for what they consider to be chiropractic's effectiveness. The spaces between the vertebrae are almost three times larger than the diameter of the spinal nerves that pass through them. (p. 64)

Benedetti and MacPhail (2002) also point out that chiropractors do not really adjust vertebrae.

Citing a research study at Yale University in 1973, where researchers

> clamped a series of fresh human spines with ligaments and spinal nerves intact, in a drill press. Using wires attached to an ohmmeter, he tested to see if the spinal nerves actually touched the edges of the foramina as he twisted and turned the spine with the controlled and measured force of the press. The results? Crelin (the main researcher in the study) couldn't stretch the spinal nerves or get the foramina to pinch or put pressure on them unless he exerted enough force to break the spine. (p. 65)

B. J. Palmer once described the manner in which a subluxation and the pressure it exerted on nerves as analogous to a person stepping on a garden hose, which would shut off the flow of water (Long, 2013). Thus, critics point out that pinched nerves caused by a subluxation is not scientifically possible, nor could the nerves be stretched or impinged as D. D. and B. J. Palmer describe. As it relates to disease, critics of sublux theory also point out that most of the nerves that relate to organs and disease are located in the skull, not in the spine, which are not manipulated by chiropractic treatments (Long, 2013).

Even members of the chiropractic profession express some concerns about how the sublux theory has continued to jeopardize their attempts at gaining credibility. As a dean of one of the chiropractic colleges noted,

We want our graduates to be able to speak the language of modern science, we want them to be critical thinkers and not be led astray by bizarre philosophies or cult-like ideas that have been a part of the old chiropractic profession. So we're wanting to make a clean split with them. And we've even gone so far as to get away from the idea of bone displacement in the spine. A lot of our fears, we call it "BOOP" around here, which stands for bone out of place. And one of our founders back in 1895, had an idea that he was putting bones back in place and that bones were pinching nerves. Of course you have to realize, he didn't even buy an anatomy book until two years after he had done the first treatment. He wasn't trained, he had no idea what he was doing, and at the time it sounded like a plausible idea . . . imagining what was going on in the spine. It didn't take long to discover that bones aren't out of place at all, and therefore the term we use, subluxation, is completely erroneous.

And this has been the source of a great deal of problems for the profession with its interactions with the medical field because when they see us using this outdated terminology like this they feel like we must believe in it and buy into these cult-like ideas as well. So we've actually restricted that we use the term that the osteopathic field uses, which is somatic dysfunction. And we call it, the subluxation, we call it the "S" word. And we only use the "S" word here when we actually and legitimately mean it as a term in its anatomical meaning. So that's the position we're taking, an evidence-based program that seeks integration with health care at large. We also put on our one-page brochure we put no longer alternative medicine. We don't want to be an alternative field. Alternative medicine implies iridology and reflexology and all those things. Chiropractic care, as a conservative form of musculoskeletal care, is about as validated as supported by literature as anything that's out there. It's far from alternative, by many standards and guidelines that have been published, it's quite mainstream.

But when guys start talking about Innate and subluxations, all the progress we've made goes out the window. Our history is important to us as a profession and we should learn the lessons from that history, and we can even celebrate it, but we have to mature as a profession and there is a faction within our group, for reasons that I just can't understand, that won't do that. I like to think people are generally reasonable and someone who has gone through doctoral level study in a scientific field should be willing to listen to reason and logically conclude that some of what we do may not make sense, but it is having an effect. The trick would be to continue to strive for an answer to that question, not simply blindly accept what someone said a hundred and twenty years ago who had a financial and legal incentive for making all sorts of wild claims.

Another observer, John, who owns a practice but is not a licensed chiropractor, offers this commentary. He says the following:

See, a lot of chiropractors talk a good game. They'll learn and use just enough medical terms and concepts to make you think they know what they're talking about. They'll even refer to books on the subject that prove how chiropractic is

> nothing more than neurophysiology and that the science of chiropractic already exists. But if you listen carefully and have even a rudimentary understanding of what's going on, you'll see it's all babble. They don't know what they're talking about—and it seems like they are simply reciting from a practice building seminar script. When you start to question them, all they know how to do is repeat what they have already said. Then again, you can't really defend something like the subluxation because they can't prove it exists. . . . But insurance companies cover it so they keep using the language that they know gets them paid.

I spent time in Joe's practice on several occasions and each time we sat down to talk about issues in the profession, a number of weeks had passed, long enough for him to have likely forgotten what he told me the last time we met. In each instance, the same explanation was offered, with the same phrases and even the same inflection of certain words used in the conversation. It almost felt as though he were reciting from a memorized script. It made me wonder if what he said to me was the same monologue he gave to his patients, some of whom are undoubtedly politely tolerant of the mantra.

Joe is clearly an advocate of the sublux theory and he goes into great detail about how to understand it. He says the following:

> I always focused on education, help your patients understand your product and that you have a unique product and why they need it. Um, why does someone need a chiropractor who does physical therapy when they can just go to a physical therapy and their insurance will pay for it? So I think that's an issue for him, he needs to understand that. That's where I get worried about our profession as we start getting swallowed up by the medics, because we want to be too much like them and we had too many guys who wanted to be medical doctors and opted to go to chiropractic college instead . . . and so because they couldn't get into med school, or because it was a little easier to get into chiropractic college, now chiropractic college is taking care of that all on its own. Now they require a four-year degree, now they are requiring a 4.0; it's not easy to get into chiropractic college, it's expensive now, so that the chiropractic colleges have done away with a lot of that.
>
> But for a long time, you had these guys, who wanted to be, what I call *Medipractors,* and they want all the rights of a medical doctor but they didn't get the medical degree. So I think those guys are in danger of watering down our profession and we are in danger of being swallowed up eventually, if we get too many guys who say, "Well, I'm just going to do physical therapy," well, all of a sudden we're practicing physical therapy, the physical therapists file a lawsuit, and eventually there could be some bad things happen. Especially guys who say that they want a proprietary drug law, we want to be able to prescribe, okay. Now we get the medical profession suing the state association in chiropractic, and pretty soon they shut the chiropractic profession down and pretty soon, our scope of practice, and we're not able to diagnose anymore.

We get that taken away from us . . . so . . . what I love about the chiropractic profession is that for a hundred and twenty years we're based on the same philosophic principles we were founded on. And that is getting the body moving. If we can restore balance, line and motion, and we can increase proprioceptive and mechanical receptive into the nervous system, that's going to shut down the stress response, that's going to shut down neuroceptive bombardment because the joint's out of alignment, that's going to normalize our physiology, it's going to normalize our catacomamines, lower cortisol, lower blood sucrose levels, all those things happen whether the medical profession wants to believe that or not. They can say it's not science, it's not quackery, it's all neurophysiology, it's been proven.

And we've got the research to prove it. But chiropractors don't seize on that. The straight chiropractors, the really philosophical guys, they're lost on that hard bone on a soft nerve. "It's a pinched nerve!" they say. That's shutting down signaling to the tissues, well, there's probably some what I call epherent component to the subluxation, but most of the physiological changes are the apherent model. . . . Um, when a joint's not firing, how it shuts down information coming into the cerebellum, where the cerebellum either reflexes back into the body or it passes information on up to the cerebrum in other areas, where it synapsed out and comes back down to the body.

That's the real beauty, and the real thing we have proven, we know that when a joint's not moving, you're compressing movement pathways. And when you compress movement pathways, you're getting garbage in and garbage out. So that's one of the things that puts the body in a state of stress and we all know fight or flight, stress response, heart rate goes up, respiration rate goes up, cholesterol levels go up, glucose levels go up, blood sugar levels go up. Everything that's killing America. So what we have to do is stay true to the principles we were founded on . . . and that's what I love about it because that's still what chiropractic is . . . regardless of what anyone will tell you, that's what it was founded on. That's what it still is today. Medicine is constantly changing, minute by minute. . . . What they were doing fifty years ago they're not doing today. What they're doing now they won't be doing in another fifty years.

[Gets up and brings back the book] Here, *The 14 Foundational Principles for the Scientific and Philosophical Validation of the Chiropractic Wellness Paradigm.* This is my bible, you can see the binding is beat up, the spine is all beat up. I use this all the time. And this book lays it out. This guy has written four books. And this guy, he's one of the only guys, that when he travels, he doesn't have to go through customs. He can show you his passport, and he's got a passport that says that he knows more about his field than anybody that resides in this country. He can walk right into any country. His name is James Chestnut.

This guy is a big deal. The Wellness Practice, that's his practice. Wait! I've got a second book here. *Global Self Help Group.* This is great, because when we go into fight or flight, the stress response, these are all the things that happen . . . increased heart rate [reads from page]. And of course there's a reason for it. . . . Why would your blood glucose go up? . . . sticky blood. Heartrate goes up . . .

> keeps reading. In the short-term that's okay, but long term not so good. When you look at chiropractic, and this is a great model. This is the neurology of the subluxation complex. It explains what happens when you have a subluxation. . . . This is the stress response here, mapped out. And that's all neurophysiology.
>
> We didn't invent this stuff. It's all the medics, it's right out of their textbooks. Okay. And so that's what I'm talking about the apherent model of chiropractic it's movement and restoring motion and the loss of motion. . . . This is how it changes your physiology. This is why people will get an adjustment and go, "geez, it helped my asthma, it helped my constipation, it helped my stomach problems." It helped my migraines. Chiropractic doesn't restore any of those, we just restore physiology. And that's what it does and then this is all backed up.
>
> So this guy is badass, he uses all the empirical references, all the physiology, all these guys and goes through the entire physiology of subluxation and what chiropractic does and this gives you the research that supports it. It's a great, great book. But I don't understand why guys aren't talking about this stuff. . . . I go to the meetings and conferences and all they want to talk about is "hey, how do you bill for this or how did you get more patients." That's not what we should be talking about—we should be talking about how the science of chiropractic is there and we just need to educate doctors and the public about what we do.

At the conclusion of this discussion, I looked for the publisher of the book and realized it was a self-published text as part of an organization that offers, among other things, practice-building seminars. I also asked many chiropractors interviewed for this project and several of the deans of chiropractic colleges around the country and no one had ever heard of this book or its author. Thus while Joe uses it as a guiding feature of his education of patients, there remain questions about whether this was a marketing script for them or a legitimate explanation of how chiropractic treatments really work.

In one of the more interesting empirical articles on vertebral subluxations, two chiropractic researchers Nanasel and Szlazak (1995) take a particular exception to the subluxation theory. They argue that if we assume the theory is correct, then people with low back pain should have greater frequency and intensity of disease in organs that are fed by the nerves coming off the spine. If this were true, Nanasel and Szlazak argue, it would be reasonable to expect that many patients suffering from this would be found in the medical literature, but that is not the case.

Additionally, they argue that if the premise on which chiropractic is based, Innate Intelligence, or the body's ability to heal itself, is valid, why does it not apply to the spine—meaning why does the spine not simply heal itself from a subluxation? The authors also ask why chiropractors are the only ones who are sufficiently gifted to treat subluxations and heal diseases? These were fascinating questions and it does not appear that the school of thought that subscribes to the Innate explanation has addressed them in any meaningful way.

One chiropractor pointed out that the notion of the Innate has other value in chiropractic medicine. He says the following:

> Some chiropractors feel that holding to, even reviving, Innate philosophy is essential to chiropractic's survival. They view Innate as the fundamental identifying principle of chiropractic, that which separates us from medicine. Innate thus serves as a guide to keep us from suffering the perceived fate of the osteopaths. To tamper with this bedrock legacy from the Palmers runs the risk of fracturing the very foundation of chiropractic. (Morgan, 1998: 38)

In discussing the doubt about subluxations in particular and chiropractic in general, Benedetti and McPhail (2002) conclude the following:

> In the end, chiropractic is left with two things: Innate, which is untestable, and the subluxation, which has not been proven to exist. In the face of that, many chiropractors simply fall back on their belief that what they do is effective, proclaiming the mantra "Chiropractic works!" (p. 79)

Instead of seeing the issue about whether or not subluxations and chiropractic medicine are legitimate, Ed, a dean of a chiropractic college, points out there may be some room for both arguments to be presented: a general disbelief of sublux theory while at the same time recognizing the value of chiropractic treatments. He says the following:

> I think spinal manipulation is a powerful tool, it's proving to be a powerful tool, but you're right. I think the theories of putting bones back in place is a little bit like Santa Claus. When you were ten you thought presents came from this guy who came down the chimney, but now we know better. I still think it is a powerful tool and is the basis of this profession. But there's tons of research coming in on the fascial system and how it feeds back into the spine. What effect are we having on the fascial system, which, again, there's a lot of sensory input, one of the guys who founded National, Joe Jensey, he was famous for saying we are sensory animals, we respond to our environment, and we do. What chiropractors are trying to do, is that sometimes our environments are overwhelming and we can't adapt quick enough and that generates these dysfunctions.
>
> So coming from an old historical perspective, they were exactly right. Now did they make up a story of what happened? Maybe, but now we know that the story, that observation, isn't changing. Yes, our sensory environment can get overwhelmed. What we are starting to understand though is exactly what's happening inside of us in terms of neuro plastic effects, feedback from the fascia system, what our nutritional status does for us. Nearly 90% of our serotonin is made in the small intestine. So what's the most common prescribed drug for depression? Things that bring up serotonin levels!

> So our argument as a chiropractor is what if we had your small intestine functioning properly, which most people's don't because the diet people have today is horrible, but if I boost your serotonin production, do you need an antidepressant? Kind of going back to the original way chiropractic works, and the theory of taking away all the interference to let the body function at an optimal level, is exactly correct. That's what we're trying to do, not as simple as taking your foot off a garden hose . . . the body's way too complicated.
>
> [You're saying we're just beginning to understand what's actually happening rather than adhering to the dogma?]
>
> It always makes me chuckle when I hear them say, "well, I'm a philosophy-based chiropractor." I'm like, no you're not, you're dogmatic. Philosophy is questions with no answers but constantly looking for the truth, you just don't know what the answer is . . . what they're saying is dogmatic, it's answers without questions. You can't question my theories because that's where they came from. Sorry, the guy who wrote it a hundred years ago . . . of course, but we're not depending on our history to guide our future. We are constantly searching for answers . . . and here's the key, what's best for our patients, what's working, what's the best response we're getting, if I can keep you off of opiates, if I can keep you off of diabetic medication, if I can keep you from meds, all good. And we're not saying medication is bad, because there's a need for it. Surgery isn't bad, because there's a need for it. But there's a lot less need for it than you actually think there is . . . it's our go-to move. . . . Whenever we have a problem we pop a pill for anything.

Interestingly, what is noted in many of the books criticizing chiropractors and the chiropractic profession is this idea that either practitioners who espouse such theories are quacks, misguided, and ignorant, or they are as deceptive and underhanded. In other words, critics of chiropractors seem to portray them either as dogmatic, who cling to unproven doctrine, or as con artists who take advantage of their victims, and offer feeble justifications and rationalizations for their actions.

It seems reasonable to conclude something is going on—perhaps in the beginning there was a bit of showmanship and a concerted effort to make a profit or to avoid a jail sentence, but what about the last one hundred years? How have chiropractors responded to these criticisms? Many opponents to the profession argue that they have not responded at all—as anti-science providers who are themselves both critical and in some cases hostile toward medicine, the chiropractic profession has not always embraced the scientific method of discovery to learn more about what they are doing and why it works.

In recent decades, many chiropractic colleges have embraced a more integrative model and attempted to learn from their perhaps colorful and questionable past. Others point out that while a fringe group of chiropractors have clung to the philosophical notions of the past despite evidence to the contrary, many in the profession have shifted their focus away from the sublux theory to a more mainstream explanation. As one dean of a chiropractic college pointed out,

> We need to celebrate our history, we need to respect our history, but we can't allow ourselves to be constrained from our history by being unwilling to examine the why part of what we are doing. It's not enough to simply say it works; it's not enough to call the Palmers geniuses and the ideas haven't changed in 120 years. Our history is important, but what's that old saying about those who don't learn from history—that they are doomed to repeat it? We are so much farther along in our understanding of what happens in the body than we were in the 1800s and dogmatic or religious fundamentalism won't cut it as an explanation for most people any longer. We need to be willing to step up and recognize that perhaps we didn't get it right the first time and we are trying to understand a very complex organism that isn't completely understood yet. That is a more reasonable approach, admitting we don't know the answers, than stubbornly following a principle because it guarantees our economic survival.

THE LIMITS OF SCIENCE AND MEDICINE

To be fair there has been some research conducted on a limited aspect of chiropractic treatment, most notably spinal manipulation for lower back pain (see, for instance, Arnold and Ehleringer, 2012; Bialosky and Bishop-Robinson, 2009; Bronfort, Haas, and Evans, 2004; Cherkin, Sherman and Devo, 2003). Criticisms of chiropractic research have centered on flawed methodological studies or ones that simply failed to show any meaningful effect. Several scholars have reviewed the methodology used in many of the studies that appear in chiropractic research journals and the general consensus is that the conclusions offered are not based on sound research protocols. This is not to say that no studies exist that demonstrate a value for chiropractic treatments, rather clinical trials and double-blind protocols that are typically used for medical research studies are lacking in those for chiropractic treatments (see, for instance, Ernst and Posadzki, 2010; Hall, 2014).

Chiropractors often respond to this criticism of the empirical data in two primary ways. First, chiropractors contend that the gold standard of scientific validity in medicine, the double-blind clinical trial, is not the only benchmark that should be used in assessing the effectiveness of chiropractic treatment. There are many ways to measure outcomes and clinical trials are but one approach. Not all data easily lends itself to a clinical trial, so the chiropractic community contends that other means of validating the effectiveness of their treatments should be considered.

Second, many chiropractors point out that medicine is not infallible in its approach to understanding disease and given that not every medical research project lends itself to clinical trials, it does not prevent medicine from drawing conclusions about a particular line of treatment. This assertion, of course, does not address the issue of the validity of vertebral subluxations, but it is worth exploring since if all medicine can be seen as limited in its understanding of disease, perhaps there is some reason to offer chiropractors some consideration in explaining the lack of understanding of the subluxation as well.

There is also something to be said about the real limits of all medicine to cure disease in that some of it must be attributed to patient compliance and the limits of science. And while there remain a group of chiropractors who continue to embrace the core foundational principles, including the existence of subluxations and chiropractic treatment for a wide assortment of diseases, some members of the profession have moved in a different direction about chiropractic's role in medicine. Not all chiropractors are content with this change, particularly those who believe that a rejection of the subluxation means a departure from the defining feature of the profession, but many chiropractors believe that commitment to the subluxation likely ensures they will remain on the fringes of the medical profession.

Most physicians would likely agree that all the answers to explaining diseases, and their causes and cures, are not known and may not ever be completely understood. Medicine is often understood as both an art and a science. The art of medicine involves some degree of interpretation and preference on how to treat certain illnesses—all providers have their own ideas about how to understand the data, what it means for their patients, and how that information informs their course of treatments for patients.

At times, physicians take a conservative approach to treating an illness even when new information is available that suggests a completely different approach is more effective. There may be good reasons for this, such as a limited number of studies with the new findings, the medical community has not adopted new guidelines that reflect this trend, or simply because there are unanswered questions about a course of treatment.

In those cases, a physician might continue to treat patients as they always have because it is medically sound and legally defensible, and there is a general understanding that one can almost always find research to support a particular position, even if they are at opposite ends of the spectrum. Above all else, medical guidelines usually maintain that clinical judgment is needed in making a decision—guidelines are not prescriptions of how to treat—they are general markers of understanding. But as a practical matter, it is not unrealistic to think that physicians simply use them to dictate what they do for all patients. This narrow view of medicine and treatment sounds a lot like what chiropractors are doing—where they do not value the research on spinal manipulation treatment, and instead use anecdotal patient feedback as an indicator of improvement of illness.

However, relieving symptoms is not necessarily the same thing as improving health or curing illnesses. Symptoms are one of the first things to disappear with any type of treatment; it is one of the reasons why physicians have great difficulty convincing patients to complete a round of antibiotics when they are fighting a cold. Patients feel better and then think they no longer need the medication. Chiropractors are also quick to point this out to patients—where a single treatment may result in less pain, but that does not mean the injury has healed.

In sum, it is fair to contend that one particular type of research study is not the only way to determine the effectiveness of a treatment—while there is great value placed on clinical trials in medicine, not all treatments easily lend themselves to such protocols. Thus, chiropractors are not completely wrong in their criticism of medicine for claiming their treatments are not scientifically proven. At the same time, however, there are reasonable limits to the use of science and the chiropractic community cannot simply produce customer satisfaction surveys, and use that data to prove chiropractic treatments improve a patient's health. Asking people if they feel better is not equivalent to them actually getting better.

As was mentioned, there is a fundamental question to be addressed about patient compliance. Whether it is a prescription for antibiotics, a regiment of physical therapy to recover from an injury, chiropractic treatments for a neck or back problem, or the success of an exercise and diet regiment, the patient is a key component to its success. What is the person or patient willing to do to get better? Are they willing to make lifestyle changes to follow a healthier diet and consistently exercise?

Are they willing to stop smoking and excessive drinking? Will they show up for their follow-up appointments and remain sufficiently disciplined to perform the exercises and activities of a treatment plan? And will they do it as a lifestyle change or only for a short period of time and then return to the behaviors that caused them to need help in the first place? Or does the person lack the ability or desire to make these changes and simply wants a pill to solve all their problems? Thus, whether they are patients of physicians, nutritionists, personal trainers, or chiropractors, the success of a given treatment pivots on the willingness of the patient to comply with the protocols. So to criticize the treatment without taking into account the willingness of the patient to complete the treatment seems unreasonable.

In short, some of the criticisms of chiropractic treatments are likely valid ones—in the absence of scientific evidence to prove that a problem exists, one has to question whether the prescribed treatment is effective. While pain is often a good marker that a problem exists, chiropractors cannot claim that such a problem is a vertebral subluxation until they can demonstrate consistently that one exists and that it is in fact causing the patient's problem. At the same time, all science, medicine included, suffers from a degree of inexactness and the human factor in the understanding of certain illnesses, diseases, and treatments influences what medical practitioners recommend and adopt as guiding principles.

These criticisms apply to chiropractors as well as to physicians. And all scientists are, to some degree, subject to personal and professional biases that color their thinking, conclusions, and behavior. This does not excuse chiropractors from being unwilling to consider the research on topics; they have an obligation and duty to understand more about what is happening in the body when an injury is sustained and how their self-identified treatments impact their patients. They also have an obligation to determine, to the extent possible, how their treatments are similar or different from other types of professions—and to acknowledge that those differences may be quite similar, in form, function, and effectiveness, to other professions' techniques in the successful treatment of back or neck pain.

They also cannot make outlandish claims to be able to heal diseases in patients without being willing to accept the criticism that comes from the lack of proof that such claims are actually valid. Chiropractors must also be willing to accept the criticisms about their profession since they are unwilling to weed out the frauds, con artists, and quacks that detract from whatever legitimate success they may have in treating people's injuries or medical problems.

IS THERE A ROLE FOR CHIROPRACTIC MEDICINE?

In addition to simply not responding to the criticisms levied against it, the chiropractic profession has an opportunity to modify the role of chiropractic medicine in health care. The opioid epidemic, as outlined by the Center for Disease Control, has provided chiropractic with an opportunity to insert itself into the discussion as a valid alternative to conventional medicine's tendency to prescribe pain killers to solve patient discomfort. As one dean of a chiropractic college pointed out, it may be that the opioid problem may cause people to begin examining the way medicine treats pain and symptoms. He says the following:

> There isn't enough conversation of the benefits of chiropractic as opposed to the danger of it. There is going to be this grass roots effort in the future. . . . And chiropractic will be at dead center of the table because of the opioid epidemic.

> So everybody, including those in the medical community, feel that chiropractic would be the first line of defense. . . . So chiropractic is getting more noted because of that epidemic. . . . It could be a saving opportunity. . . . Drugs save lives, but that creates a moral panic about what are we going to do differently for people who needed surgery. . . . Do they need it in the first place? If you could knock the opioid addiction by 50% you'd save thousands of lives and millions of dollars. . . . So there's a grass roots effort that people are becoming educated about their health. . . . Once I have heart problems I'm always going to have heart problems, so people are taking vitamins and exercising and eating better. So as people take responsibility for their own health, including preventative measures, the outlook is more positive.

According to a recent statement by the American College of Physicians, non-drug treatments should be used as a guiding principle to treat something like lower back pain before using medications. This is heralded to be a significant departure from conventional medicine's stance in the past, where rest and non-prescription strength pain medications were considered the most appropriate way to handle something like low back pain (Qassem et al., 2017). The following are the three primary recommendations from the organization:

Recommendation 1: Given that most patients with acute or subacute low back pain improve over time regardless of treatment, clinicians and patients should select non-pharmacologic treatment with superficial heat (moderate-quality evidence), massage, acupuncture, or spinal manipulation (low-quality evidence). If pharmacologic treatment is desired, clinicians and patients should select nonsteroidal anti-inflammatory drugs or skeletal muscle relaxants (moderate-quality evidence).

Recommendation 2: For patients with chronic low back pain, clinicians and patients should initially select non-pharmacologic treatment with exercise, multidisciplinary rehabilitation, acupuncture, mindfulness-based stress reduction (moderate-quality evidence), tai chi, yoga, motor control exercise, progressive relaxation, electromyography biofeedback, low-level laser therapy, operant therapy, cognitive behavioral therapy, or spinal manipulation (low-quality evidence).

Recommendation 3: In patients with chronic low back pain, who have had an inadequate response to non-pharmacologic therapy, clinicians and patients should consider pharmacologic treatment with nonsteroidal anti-inflammatory drugs as first-line therapy, or tramadol or duloxetine as second-line therapy. Clinicians should only consider opioids as an option in patients who have failed the aforementioned treatments and only if the potential benefits outweigh the risks for individual patients and after a discussion of known risks and realistic benefits with patients (Qaseem et al., 2017).

Notice that this statement is not an endorsement of chiropractic treatment. The recommendations point out that most patients with back pain improve over time regardless of the type of treatment they receive, including doing nothing. It also points out that there is low-quality evidence of the effectiveness of some treatments, including spinal manipulation.

Rather, these guidelines suggest that less invasive remedies have fewer long-term consequences and should be used initially when a patient experiences a problem, such as lower back pain. This does not, by itself, suggest chiropractic treatments are called for, although the statement does not exclude them as one of several possible remedies (Qaseem et al., 2017; see also Ciccone, 2017).

These guidelines, along with a video testimonial about them, were recently included on the American Chiropractic Association's (ACA) website. The implication, of course, is that the guidelines validate spinal manipulation as a form of treatment. That is a debatable interpretation, but what is perhaps even more interesting is that there is no mention of vertebral subluxation either in the video, the guidelines, or even on the entire ACA website.

What is discussed are the problems relating to lower back pain, headaches, and other ailments and the role of spinal manipulation in treating those problems. In fact, the research identified on the website, as well as from other websites, blogs, and other sources, points to musculoskeletal problems, typically focused on the lower back and the neck, and the consistently limited level of success in treating these ailments with spinal manipulation.

To be fair, much of the research on this topic is rather equivocal: the findings tend to show that spinal manipulation is one of several different treatment options available and there is usually some notation that the treatment is either mildly effective or no more effective than other forms of treatment, including doing nothing at all (Qaseem et al., 2017). Thus, the language and the narrative appear to have shifted away from the vertebral subluxation as a centerpiece of the chiropractic treatment. This is particularly true given that the ACA is the largest chiropractic organization in the world.

While the ACA has moved away from defending vertebral subluxations as a key component to the chiropractic paradigm, not all chiropractic organizations have done so. The International Chiropractic Association, along with the Federation of Straight Chiropractors, has embraced the original core principles that adhere to the idea that vertebral subluxations exist, that the reduction of these subluxations can be identified through x-rays, and that the relief of subluxations cures disease and can only be performed by chiropractors.

A review of that website indicates an effort to legitimize this portion of the profession by creating a set of guidelines for treatment, an attempt to review the available research on the success of chiropractic adjustments, as well as addressing some of the limitations of the current wave of research on the subject. In fact, a significant portion of the guidelines includes a lengthy discussion of research methodology concepts and a criticism of clinical trials as a form of research in chiropractic medicine. In its place, there is a greater emphasis on qualitative research to assess the impact of chiropractic treatment.

SCOPE OF PRACTICE: STRAIGHTS, MIXERS, AND REFORMERS

As was mentioned, part of the challenge of understanding chiropractor's scope of practice, either in general or in a particular state, begins with how chiropractors see themselves. In some cases, chiropractors adhere to strictly defined principles that focus on subluxations and adjustments that cure disease. This group also tends to adopt the notion of the Innate and the body's ability to heal itself. Chiropractors in this category are often referred to as *Straights* or straight chiropractors.

This group tends to take a narrow view of what chiropractors should be doing and think chiropractors should not be doing anything other than adjustments. These types of chiropractors tend to affiliate with the International Chiropractic Association or the Federation of Straight Chiropractors and eschew notions of expanding the profession beyond its original principles. Topics such as prescription drug laws are considered to be outside the scope of practice for these providers. As Joe points out, the problem with something like prescription drug laws is that it tends to blur the identity of the profession. He says the following:

> So a lot of schools, like National, and these guys are working really hard for the proprietary drug laws, basically, they just want the money. And they're going for laws they might try for an adjustment, but if you got something going on, they're going to prescribe a muscle relaxer or pain pill, and pretty soon, chiropractors are just a general practitioner and he's just a referral station. And we don't need that. And these guys are what I call Meta-practors, they're guys that want to have prescription and proprietary drug laws, where they can prescribe muscle relaxers and pain pills. That's the last thing we need in this country is somebody else doling out a pill. We don't. We're the most medicated country in the world. One country takes 68% of all the medication in the world. The United States does. The only country, out of what, 237 something countries, or whatever it is? We take 68% of the meds. So we're the most overmedicated country in the world but yet, if medication really worked, we'd be the healthiest nation in the world, but we're not. We're like 74th on the World Health Organization's list. What we're doing isn't working. That's like I talk to people about cholesterol and blood pressure medication all the

> time. I say the highest killers of Americans, the number one is heart disease. That's what they're giving you blood pressure and cholesterol medication for. Last year, we had more people than ever before taking blood pressure and statin drugs, but the heart disease rate still continued to rise. If this were working, we'd see this going down. It's not working. People are just dying with better numbers. People have better numbers but they are still dying of heart disease because we're not getting to the root cause of why we're developing all these meds.

Mike, a dean at a chiropractic college had this to say about prescription drug laws:

> I think you're starting to see . . . prescription drugs are a mistake. And when you ask the public, they're not thinking about going to a chiropractor for a prescription. The Gallup polls show that. There's a specific reason they're going to a chiropractor. . . . They don't want to take a pill; they want a different alternative. I think prescription rights is a mistake for the profession. . . . We're not going to legitimize ourselves by having prescription drug rights. That's not what the patient is looking for though. The other aspect of this, we saw the ACA, which is the broadest representative of chiropractic, in their 2017 conference in DC, they are finally taking a stand--this is what chiropractic is to us, which is primary care spine specialists conservative care, drugless or surgery, and looking for evidence formed solutions to patient care. That was a big stand for the ACA, because for years they tried to be inclusive to everybody, now they are saying here's who we are and if you don't agree with it, there's other associations. I think we might be starting to turn a corner on that because our national association is starting to find what chiropractic should be . . . not being all-inclusive in order to get on the same page. I will tell you, if you put two chiropractors in a room and you'll have about 20 different opinions.

In contrast to straights are chiropractors known as *Mixers*, who integrate other types of treatments with chiropractic medicine. This group would be more likely to recognize that they cannot solve every patient's health problem through chiropractic treatments and would be more likely to refer a patient to a physician or specialist if their situation called for it. As Kat points out,

> I personally have a lot of friends, especially sports chiropractors who are definitely working with soft tissue and muscle, as opposed to joints. I mean, I prefer to be a subluxation-based chiropractor, I like adjusting people and think it works well by itself. If they need something else, I don't think chiropractic fixes everything automatically. I think it depends on how they have been injured or how long they've been injured, how chronic their condition is, they could need other types of treatment. . . . They could need soft tissue work, they could need

> massage, and in certain cases they'll need surgery or injections. But I feel like we're sort of like portal of entry in terms of orthopedic type conditions. . . . and subluxation-based chiropractic is just adjusting the easiest way to start and that's what I like to focus on. And a lot of times it is effective and they don't need to do anything else.

This group, which obviously includes a wider spectrum of providers who believe in various treatments for patients, also tends to include treatments such as nutritional supplements, weight loss, and other modalities, such as acupuncture. However, many tend to agree with straight chiropractors in that they generally believe in the sublux theory and that chiropractic should not be limited only to neck and back issues. Some disagree with the sublux theory, but there lacks the consistency of agreement found among Straights. Doug, who says he's a straight chiropractor, says he has been accused of being a Mixer because he offers nutritional supplements, and explains his understanding of how it works. He says the following:

> The body is designed as a self-healing, self-regulating organism and that the way the body regulates that is through functioning of the central nervous system, the brain, the spinal column and the associated spinal nerves. That's where chiropractic comes in. Because we have so many stressors that we're subject to, we have three types of stressors that we're exposed to: Physical Stressors, Chemical Stressors and Emotional Stressors. And the thing about the body is that it doesn't distinguish among stressors, it just recognizes stress. And so the body reacts the same way every time: that sympathetic dominance; fight or flight system. That system is built into us from the beginning of time. And it's a great system have because it can save our lives. The problem is, we're designed to have that system activated about 10–15 minutes at a time. You go to the water hole; you encounter a saber tooth tiger. You got one choice, you gotta fight or you gotta run. Fight or flight. So you go into that sympathetic dominance, fight of flight system, heart rate goes up, respiration rate goes up. . . . Blood glucose levels go up. Blood becomes sticky. Your ability to learn algebra is shut down; you're like this because you gotta be looking around. That's fight or flight. Okay?
>
> Short-term those are all good things. Long-term, not good to have high heart rate, not good to have high respiration rate; high blood pressure. Sticky blood. Why would your blood become sticky? Because if you're in a fight or flight situation and you get cut, good to have sticky blood. Okay? Why does your heart rate go up? Well, you've got to oxygenate those muscles so you can be strong and you can run fast. Same thing for your respiration rate—why would your blood glucose level go up? Because glucose is energy, body need that to burn right away. You don't have time to go into ketosis and break down fat. So all those things short-term are good.

But because we have so many stressors . . . chemicals in the foods we eat, preservatives, the perfumes, roll-ons, the additives, the cleaning, the fabrics, everything. That's a huge stressor for us. Environmental chemicals . . . physical stressors, we sit at a desk all day, we sit in a car that's not designed properly. People doing the same jobs over and over, lots of micro-traumas, those are physical stressors. And then there's emotional stressors; pissed off at my kids, pissed off at my wife, pissed off at my job, not happy with this, not happy with that, we don't have ways to deal with that. We carry that with us all day. So now our sympathetic nervous system is dominated 24 hours a day—it's on. So that's one of the things that's contributing to the heart disease, stroke, cancer, it's a stress response we're stuck in. That's what chiropractic does.

We start firing off those movement pathways; we start relieving the pressure on the central nervous system and we allow our body to start to get into a relaxed state. It regulates our physiology so I think that when chiropractors come in and say, "Doc, I think I've got a pinched nerve." Well, you probably do, but there's probably not a hard bone on a nerve, there's probably happening is something's moved out of place, the joint's not firing properly anymore. That's creating some swelling and some pressure around the nerve root, and it could be causing some pain. But what we've done is we've shut down the functioning of those movement pathways, and those movement pathways are the learning pathways. They're the pathways that are the relaxation pathways; they're the pathways that when they're firing, you're inhibiting the stress pathways. Because your body can't be in a state of relaxation and a state of stress at the same time. You're doing one or the other. So what we're doing is we're stimulating that exchange of information between the brain and the body, we're flooding the cerebellum with proprioceptive input, and that's what shuts down those stress pathways and allows your body to get back into a relaxed state. And so for years chiropractic has focused on the hard bone on a soft nerve, pinching. Well that probably does happen, we just can't prove it. but we do know what happens to those afferent pathways coming back into the brain, we know that the ultimate goal of the brain is to find out what the body's needs are what the body's doing. So the brain can respond and regulate physiology. Garbage in garbage out, so we got to have those pathways gathering information so the brain can either send it to the cerebellum and process that information, higher critical thinking, memorization, things like that require higher levels of the brain, that will get shipped up to the brain and then the brain will deal with it. But most of it is handled right there at the brain stem. That's basically what the principle of chiropractic is all about. . . . Just basically, creating a solid foundation for the body to function properly, clear that nervous system out for communication and the body will go towards a state of homeostasis.

Finally, there are *Reformers*. This group tends to view chiropractic medicine as part of a larger integrative model, where chiropractors are part of a larger collaborative medical team. Reformers tend to view the history of chiropractic with disdain and sharply disagree with many of the basic principles of the profession such as sublux theory and Innate. They would like chiropractors to be viewed as primary care physicians and the training they receive tends to be more along the lines of what medical students obtain in medical school.

Reformers also tend to focus on the value of chiropractic medicine as a first line of defense in the treatment of patients, where they can resolve a host of problems before a patient needs to see a specialist. Given that they are collaborative, who work closely with physicians, physical therapists, massage therapists, and other medical providers, they tend to see their contributions as part of a larger collective whole. They also tend to view the scope of practice for chiropractors beyond simply treating neck or back injuries, although that is their specialty. As Tom, a dean at one of the chiropractic colleges noted,

> So I think most schools have jumped on to being more of a primary care spine specialist. Patients are coming to us because of spinal complaints. That's what brings 90% of patients into a chiropractor's office. If a patient is coming to us for nutritional counseling, they've been to a chiropractor before and they know they do nutritional counseling. And I think what the schools are trying to do is latch on to what the public wants and thinks we do . . . and how to they see us and how do we prepare students to get them ready to serve them based on how they see us. I mean, we as chiropractors can say all day long what we think we should be doing, we are effective in treating Irritable Bowel Syndrome, we are effective at treating migraines, but if you have Irritable Bowel Syndrome, we're not your first thought.
>
> Now, eventually, you may get to us, and we might be effective in treating it, but we're not your first thought. So I think a lot of schools are moving much more towards that. *JAMA* [Journal of the American Medical Association] just published an article that says spinal manipulation therapy is effective in dealing with back pain, which is a huge thing for us because for the longest time *JAMA* has been dead set against chiropractic. Partially it's our own fault though because we weren't providing the evidence. Now we are starting to provide the evidence, they did a Cochran review and all of a sudden, we're popping up and people are starting to say "Hey maybe these guys aren't as crazy as we thought they were." . . . I think that's the maturing process. . . . We realize what we have to do. A lot of the knocks against us are our own fault. To be fair it's not our fault that we didn't have data for 120 years. I can't manufacture it. And you can't generate data when all the research institutions say we're not going to work with you. How do we get there then? And where is the funding coming from? We can't just prove it on a dime, nor can we get it right away.

There are many chiropractors who are a blend of each group and may agree with one school of thought on a particular issue, but disagree with them in other areas. As one dean of a chiropractic college points out, it can be a bit confusing, particularly as this debate impacts how a particular college trains its students. The politics involved sometimes causes colleges to avoid any type of self-labeling out of fear of upsetting alumni from that institution.

> There are some schools that are very clear in their orientations, and others that are on the fence and are afraid to go one way or the other because they are afraid to upset their alumni, a very sensitive thing, as you discovered, there really are two professions not one. There's the chiropractic profession, very vitalistic, and stuck in its baggage of the past, as evidenced by Sherman College for example, and then there's chiropractic medicine, a very progressive shield that seeks to be very integrated with conventional healthcare and that's the approach we're taking here.
>
> I've been in chiropractic education for 21 years now and I've seen the challenges from schools that are sitting on the fence. For example, at Northwestern Health Sciences University in Minnesota, they are so afraid of their alumni it's ridiculous. These are a fraction of the population and they only pay fifty dollars a year and they are so afraid of upsetting them they are afraid to do anything.
>
> There are very few colleges that are willing to go out there. . . . Los Angeles is one, Keiser and National University are others and on the other side of the fence you have Life, Cleveland, and Sherman. And Life West. Our graduates can earn the trust of others in the healthcare fields, and we want them to be able to speak the language of modern science, we want them to be critical thinkers and not be led astray by bizarre philosophies or cult like ideas that have been a part of the old chiropractic profession. So we're wanting to make a clean split with them.

There is also a good bit of animosity between Straights, Mixers, and Reformers, as each believes theirs is the most appropriate method of presenting chiropractic medicine to the public and to the medical community. While Reformers tend to see Straights as cult-like and dogmatic, Straights tend to see Mixers as those who are not being true to their professional roots and risk diluting the profession to the point where it has not identity at all. As Doug points out,

> I think the rift between the groups is causing more harm to the profession, quite honestly. Straight chiropractors see things in black and white while the Mixers tend to see the fact that this bone on a nerve model isn't really defensible, so they're trying to take a more holistic approach just so that we remain relevant in the conversation. But Mixers think Straights are nuts and Straights think Mixers are diluting the profession and are traitors to the cause. And Reformers? Nobody seems to know what to do with those guys because they want to think of themselves as M.D.s and are practicing like doctors.

Kathleen talks about her experiences coming to South Carolina from Illinois, where she had little exposure to the straight chiropractic influence. The dogmatic approach was counter to anything she had experienced in her training or exposure to other chiropractors. She says the following:

> It's a little strange, I understand they want us to know that information and I appreciate the education, absolutely, but it's in most states most of those things are not within our scope of practice so we see it in school, we learn how to do it, but then we never see it again. Which, I can see why they would want us to have that education because we are working on the human body, but again, my school specifically lost sight of the philosophy of chiropractic and just the bread and butter part of chiropractic. . . . So for me that was difficult coming out of school because my education was completely different, I feel, than most chiropractors around here.
>
> And scope of practice in Illinois is a lot bigger and in other states is a lot bigger. So if I was in Illinois right now I could, other than writing prescriptions and doing surgery, I could be a primary care doctor. And that's National's philosophy, is they are teaching you how to be a primary care doctor. They want to follow the path of Osteopaths. Where I can see where that could be beneficial . . . I mean I wouldn't mind having limited prescription rights, for mild pain killer, muscle relaxers, which means I wouldn't have to send my patients somewhere else, which is kind of a pain, I mean that would be helpful. But full prescription rights? I mean, no. I don't have any business prescribing benzos or antibiotics or anything like that. But the more mild stuff, for muscle pain, that's fine.
>
> [But isn't it a class of drugs? So if you're able to prescribe for muscle relaxants, can't you then also prescribe to do antidepressants, is that the rub?]
>
> Right, that is part of the issue. And again, too it would depend on an opiate painkiller versus a non-opiate painkiller. I don't think any chiropractor, especially not myself, would want to prescribe any opiate or any narcotic . . . just some of the steroidal or anti-inflammatories.

While many chiropractors are beginning to use the language of an evidence-based or an evidence-informed approach to what they do, because there has not been a great deal of quality research on the effectiveness of chiropractic treatments, they are drawing from other professions and their techniques to validate chiropractic. For example, many chiropractors refer to techniques used in physical therapy, which have been scientifically validated over the years, to justify the use of particular treatments by chiropractors. As Kat points out,

> Well they don't have a lot of data about chiropractic. It isn't necessarily based on studies for chiropractic in particular, but they teach you more about how to read studies, how to process all that information and how to use like, hard to explain . . . how to use information from, say, different specialties that pertain to the kind of thing you're doing and use that information to make an educated decision about the kind of treatment you want to give your patient. Because

there are a lot of, like in PT, they do a lot of chiropractic-type treatments that are given a different name because they are physical therapists and so we can use that just as a way to make an informed decision.

[Okay, so that's what they mean by evidenced-based, by looking at the things someone else has done and has been empirically validated?]

Right, and also like, just teaching students how to actually speak that language, so you can communicate with other people who want that kind of evidence.

[So would you say . . . that the evidence-based group are much more likely to be willing to acknowledge the value of research, in that "Hey we just learned that this kind of adjustment works better than that type of adjustment and here's the data that proves that" . . . as opposed to the more philosophical folks that are going back to innate intelligence and Palmer scope, they're not as interested in the research component to it, so it's not an anti-research stance?]

I mean it's . . . I don't know, to me, it's almost . . . in certain realms of chiropractic, there's almost a religious aspect to it, that I'm really uncomfortable with actually. And I do think that's the case with that kind of lean in your education. I mean I personally, and all of the classmates that I know, they're really interested in like finding out what's new and what kind of new, like new PT techniques you can use, and there are a lot of PT modalities in the clinic. But I think that's just the nature of anyone who's done research, I think you just understand better and more about science in general and how there needs to be very little ego in it. As opposed to "I'm right, this is right, this is our philosophy and that's it."

I do a lot of stuff that just works in certain areas, just based on experience . . . kids especially . . . like when you adjust babies in a certain way it is almost always if they're constipated and it fixes that or certain adjustments will result in the baby being less colicky. And it's like, very consistent. Something you do over and over again. And I don't know why it works and I don't have any data on it, and because the procedures or techniques themselves are so non-invasive, I don't feel uncomfortable using them on people, because I don't feel like I'm putting anyone in danger just because I don't know how it works exactly.

This division within the profession between Straights, Mixers, and Reformers is seen in the inconsistency among states with regard to their stated scope of practice. While some states are quite liberal in what they allow chiropractors to do, other states narrowly define the range of activities for chiropractors. In Illinois, for example, chiropractors are allowed virtually the same rights as physicians, with two notable exceptions: prescription authorization and performing surgery. According to the website from the Illinois Chiropractic Society, the Medical Practices Act of 2011, the following identifies the scope of practice for chiropractors.

The Illinois Medical Practice Act (MPA) is one of many licensure acts within the State of Illinois. There are over 20 professional acts within the healthcare field alone (including massage therapists, dentists, physicians). The MPA is the primary law that governs the physicians in our state by defining our scope, requirements for licensure, and guidelines for discipline.

Illinois is unique in that chiropractic physicians are covered under the very same act that licenses medical doctors and doctors of osteopathic. This gives us an extra advantage when arguing for equality at the statehouse because in Illinois under the MPA DCs are statutorily defined as physicians:

"Physician" means a person licensed under the Medical Practice Act to practice medicine in all of its branches or a chiropractic physician.

The MPA further defines chiropractic physicians (this is often referred to as our scope of practice):

"Chiropractic physician," means a person licensed to treat human ailments without the use of drugs and without operative surgery. Nothing in this Act shall be construed to prohibit a chiropractic physician from providing advice regarding the use of non-prescription products or from administering atmospheric oxygen. Nothing in this Act shall be construed to authorize a chiropractic physician to prescribe drugs. (Illinois Chiropractic Society, 2012)

As the Society's website explains,

The Act in no way defines nor restricts the types of ailments or conditions which may or may not be treated by chiropractic physicians. Furthermore, it clarifies that chiropractic physicians are not prohibited from advising the use of non-prescription products (such as over-the-counter drugs) or atmospheric oxygen (oxygen concentrators, hyperbaric chambers). (Illinois Chiropractic Society, 2012)

Essentially then, a chiropractor in Illinois is authorized to conduct gynecological exams, draw blood, take x-rays, and do anything short of prescribing drugs or performing surgery. One wonders if an average patient would think of going to a chiropractor as a primary care physician, but in that state, a chiropractor can do almost everything a physician might do.

In contrast, according to the laws of South Carolina, the scope of practice for chiropractors tends to be limited to a narrower range of activities typically associated with traditional chiropractic treatment. According to the state's Department of Labor, Licensing and Regulation the scope of practice is as follows:

Persons licensed by the Board shall be limited in their practice to the care and performance of therapeutic treatment of patients, the performance of such procedures as are normally followed in giving chiropractic physical examinations,

> the x-ray of patient and such other procedures as are generally used in the practice of chiropractic.
>
> Such other procedures as are generally used in the practice of chiropractic shall be limited, however, to the use of diagnostic and therapeutic procedures, the adjustment and manipulation of articulations and treatment of inter-segmental disorders for alleviation of related neurological aberrations.
>
> Patient care shall be conducted with due regard for environmental, hygiene, sanitation, rehabilitation and physiological therapeutic procedures designed to assist in the restoration and maintenance of neurological integrity of the nervous system. None of these diagnostic or therapeutic procedures shall include the use of drugs, surgery, cauterization, desiccation or coagulation of tissues, rectal examinations, gynecological examinations, obstetrics, catheterization with a needle, injecting of dyes for radiological procedures, lumbar puncture to obtain spinal fluid, treatment of cancer or x-ray therapy. (South Carolina Department of Labor, Licensure and Regulation, 2017)

Despite prescribed ranges of activities, even a narrow definition like that outlined in the South Carolina statutes does not completely protect patients from questionable treatments by some chiropractors. One example involves whether patients need regular visits or maintenance therapy to remain in good health.

SCOPE OF PRACTICE AND MAINTENANCE THERAPY

One's training at a particular chiropractic college and its philosophy, the state's legal parameters of scope of practice, along with their individual views of the profession (whether they see themselves as Straight, Mixer, or Reformer), all influence a chiropractor's philosophy of treatment. This is particularly evident when one considers the issue of maintenance therapy. Some chiropractors believe, for example, that patients should come to see them only when they have sustained an injury. Their role as providers is to address the problem, provide treatment, and get the patient back to their level of activity as quickly as possible with a minimum number of visits to the office. As Kathleen says:

> So a lot of the chiropractors are doing the same thing. . . . And some of that debate I think revolves around money. . . . I don't think it's that we really believe as much that they need maintenance as they like having them coming in regularly and paying $50 every time they come in . . . and it's not really hurting the patients to do that . . . so is it wrong? But you don't go to physical therapy once a week for the rest of your life. You go to physical therapy for six weeks, eight weeks and you're better. I don't like people coming in for rest of their life.

Maybe if a guy has a manual labor job, and they may need regular adjustment or once a month, but for most people? No.

[But I get the idea because if you have that kind of job where you are doing something physically demanding, those are re-sustained injuries. . . . It's not maintenance, it's that I reinjured myself with my lifestyle or my activities.] Exactly. So those are different kinds of episodes, not because your joint is flowing and the Innate is working. . . . I can get the idea behind the notion of injuries and they are healed. So you go back to your specialist and you have surgery or you manage this on your own. . . . But that's different from feeling like you're working me to get money out of me. That's a huge issue in the profession.

And I don't know how many you've talked to but I know a lot of guys who do this initial consult and this work up with x-rays and a report with the binders and that you're going to die. . . . I'm going to make you come in 40 times in the next six months and it's going to cost you $2,500. . . . How come every single person who walks in the door is doing the same prescription? If it was a different kind of injury . . . and the lack of curvature in your neck is about 90% of the population and it's not that big of a deal. You can't. There's been no studies that have shown you can cure that curve with adjustment. Structurally . . . I mean you can work on the muscles and there are certain exercises that you can do to help, but structurally you can't change the structure of the spine with chiropractic adjustment. . . . But if I said that to my colleagues? Oh my god! I'd get lynched.

Tom, a dean at one of the chiropractic colleges in the United States, had this to say about the notion of maintenance therapy:

The ultimate goal where health care has moved towards is patient responsibility. You know if you take care of yourself, you eat right, exercise, you're going to take care of a lot of issues that are popping up. The problem in medicine that has been prevalent for a long time is that we'll take care of you. Well, no, take care of yourself. That's also an issue in chiropractic. . . . There are some practice management firms that push you to say, make sure your patient keeps coming in because if they keep coming in you'll keep them healthy. . . . Boy, that's the wrong message to send. We have to turn the cure back over to you. What chiropractors have to realize is you're not keeping them healthy, they're keeping themselves healthy, now if they are exercising on a regular basis, guess what's going to happen? Their back is going to hurt; their knee is going to hurt. Because they're active. Active people have more musculoskeletal complaints. We're the people to come to for that because we're not going to use drugs, we're not going to use surgery, we're going to fix this by finding the mechanical dysfunction and correct it so you can get back out there exercising again.

That's where seeing us on a regular basis is helpful. It's to keep you active. We're not saying, and there's models out there like that Bob, we're not going to say they're aren't, there are guys out there who say see me three times a week for the rest of your life and you'll never get sick again, well, that's a lie. There's no evidence for that, there's no evidence that prophylactic spinal manipulation does anything to make a patient feel better. Now if a patient likes coming in, and they say they feel better when they get adjusted regularly, can I come in on a regular basis? Sure! But I'm not going to charge insurance because that's wellness care.

So it's . . . we just need to mature more as a profession and asking what are we exactly doing and what is our acute care strategies, our chronic care strategies, what is our wellness care strategies? Most of the things we try to teach our students here is to get your patients to wellness care where they have an active lifestyle. . . . You're not going to lose them because they're active, they're going to get hurt, they're going to come in again. Or, if they're not active, they're going to get lazy, they're going to start slipping and they'll be back in again to get active again. We keep perpetuating that as an idea.

[But then there are those guys who say, no, I need to keep the joint flowing, I need to keep the Innate moving, you need to be here.] There is absolutely no evidence for that, despite the fact that they swear by it. And they get their patients to believe they need to buy the certain number of visits for a particular amount of money. That's the dogmatic approach. . . . I mean, you come into my office for 54 visits and you go get two Big Macs, a couple of milkshakes and you're sitting on the couch a lot, I mean, really? That's not working.

In contrast, other chiropractors view regular visits as an important part of their overall wellness plan. These chiropractors believe that in order to remain healthy, patients need to come to the office for treatment on a regular basis, more often if they have sustained an injury. As Joe points out,

[What about those chiropractors who say they only should be treating patient when the patient needs an adjustment? I see the muscle relaxers on the shelves. . . . Do they know what or who they are?]

No I don't think they do, I think they're confused. And to me, the ultimate goal is to get the patient out of the office as quickly as possible. I get that. You have to help the patient understand why they need you and why they need to be there. At look, you sit at a computer eight hours a day. And if you sit like this, your posture is going to break down over twenty years. Well, neurophysiology shows that every physiological function in your body is closely dictated by your posture. Loss of the thoracic clitosis, increases the loss of lung capacity by 30%, so I'm not saying you need to be here three times a week, I'm just saying you need to be here three times a week in the beginning because what we're trying to do is retrain those neural pathways that become neuroplastic. It's just like a muscle, a muscle atrophies if you put a cast on it. What do you have to do to get that muscle back? You gotta work it . . . nerves are the same way. When joints stop moving, the neural pathways associated with that joint function stop firing. They become neural plastic.

When we start adjusting you, we start reactivating those neural pathways, we get them firing, we get them firing, pretty soon we break down that neuroplasticity and they're working. That takes repetition over time. So you might have to come in three times a week for four weeks and then two times a week for four weeks, and then we'll go into what I call maintenance, maybe once a week for a couple of weeks, and after about 60–90 days, we've reactivated those pathways, we've got those joints healthy again, we've restored movement, now if you go back to doing the same thing over and over again, and you never take care of it again, we're starting over again in three or four years.

But if you come once a month, we can maintain the work that we've done. Just like, you lost all that weight, you can't go back to eating the way you did before. You don't have to be on negative calorie intake because you're trying to lose, you're able to loosen up your diet a little bit, but you still need to eat right to maintain. Same thing for exercise. You got in shape so you can run the breast cancer awareness race. Now if you run twice a week, next year you don't have to train for the race. But if you stop running all together, you got to start all over and you have to start training about twelve weeks out to get ready for that race.

So maintenance is not new to chiropractic, it's been around forever. So that's what I try to help my patients understand. I want you to feel better. And you're gonna start to feel better after about four or five adjustments. But here's why you don't want to quit. Because symptoms are always the last thing to show up in a health condition, and they're the first thing to go away.

So that's what I try to help people understand. So I give my patients those options, I say, if you want to use chiropractic as like a pain pill or muscle relaxant for temporary pain relief, you can do that and I'm happy to help you with that. Just understand that this is what you're doing and over time this problem will progress and get worse. If you want to correct it, we can do that too, you have the choice, here's the information, you make an informed decision.

Dave had this to say about maintenance therapy:

I understand the argument that some chiropractors use to justify maintenance therapy. What they basically say is that as long as you use the term "medically necessary" you are going to get reimbursed for it. So instead of calling it maintenance therapy, which won't be covered by insurance, and I'm not sure why, they game the system and say it is a new injury or an aggravation of one that happened a while ago. So the argument is like, "hey you are sitting a certain way at a desk for a long period of time each day or you are doing something that causes your posture to be poor so you get a back ache or neck pain." Some chiropractors will classify this as a "new" injury. And I get that to some extent. If you're doing the same thing over and over again that caused an injury at one point, it's likely that it will cause it again too. Football players, especially running backs, get hammered every Sunday, so many of them will be treated by chiropractors. But that's not maintenance therapy. Maintenance therapy is something the philosophical guys buy into because they think, like brushing your teeth every day, it is preventative of other problems. Other guys become convinced maintenance therapy is important because some practice building seminar idiot told them that's a way of making sure you have steady income.

> So they justify it using the philosophical ideology, but that seems underhanded to me. . . . You don't really believe in the treatment, it is nothing more than churning patients. And some patients will buy into it, and that's okay. But you are going to get chiropractic treatments for your back and neck for the rest of your life? Come on. That is not medically necessary.

What is interesting about the use of maintenance therapy is that it is not covered under most insurance plans. While Medicare and other insurance plans have placed a yearly limit on the number of visits, these are intended to be used for particular injuries sustained by a patient during the year. But insurance does not reimburse for regular visits to maintain a patient's health. This has a number of consequences for chiropractors and for patients. One of those is that chiropractors have to manage patients' expectations about the cost. They must convince patients that they actually need further treatment even though their patients must pay for it out of pocket. As Brad points out,

> And then you have to tell the patients they have to pay after four visits. . . . In the very beginning it was a lot more difficult because it was a lot more difficult. And I am not sure it was because I wasn't as confident in telling the patients. . . . Here's what your insurance is going to cover, or it's because insurance in the four and a half years since I've been here has changed quite dramatically, um, at this point patients are . . . you know, if I say to patients "this is what your insurance is going to cover," a lot of them kind of roll their eyes . . . or a lot of times we say your contract says it's this and the difference is $52, my time of service if you are paying without insurance we can bill you forty dollars. But it is hard to convince patients that what I'm doing is nothing more than what the insurance company is allowing me to do. . . . The patient has to decide if they want to pay for my services out of pocket. But a lot of times they think I'm just trying to take advantage of them and I'm really not. I'm just telling them what the insurance plan they're on covers. They can decide what to do next.

Another issue is that chiropractors often attempt to submit invoices for services to insurance companies even though they know that the plan does not cover maintenance therapy. As a result, many insurance carriers have begun to audit chiropractors in an attempt to force them to justify the treatments provided as medically necessary and not maintenance. A recent report by the Office of Inspector General, a division of the Department of Health and Human Services, revealed that a large portion of the inappropriate Medicare billing comes from chiropractors (Office of Inspector General, 2017).

Because the fees amount to millions of dollars each year, Medicare has instituted accountability measures using algorithms to determine if a provider is excessively billing the system. The result has been that some chiropractors were formally audited by Medicare and the fines and penalties for misleading information or fraud are significant. It also requires chiropractors to pay back reimbursement fees if the audit determines the treatment to be more of a maintenance one than a new injury. Because this is a significant problem, with millions of dollars at stake, this topic will be covered in more depth in the chapter on health care reform.

TEXAS AND SCOPE OF PRACTICE

The issue and controversy over chiropractors' scope of practice has been a common point of contention in Texas, where the Texas Medical Association (TMA) has taken issue with many treatments conducted by chiropractors. In September 2006, the Medical Association filed a lawsuit against the Texas Board of Chiropractic Examiners, the entity that oversees licensure of chiropractors. The basis of this lawsuit was that the Board allowed chiropractors to perform a treatment called needle electromyography (EMG), as well as allowing chiropractors to perform spinal manipulation on patients under anesthesia (MUA).

According to the American Academy of Family Physicians, EMG is an invasive process where a thin needle is inserted into the patient to measure the muscles' electrical activity. This procedure is used to diagnose illnesses such as Lou Gehrig's disease and carpel tunnel syndrome. It remains controversial, largely as it relates to which types of medical providers should be allowed to conduct this test and whether it can be used as a diagnostic or treatment tool (American Academy of Family Physicians, 2017).

The TMA amended the lawsuit to challenge chiropractors' ability to render any diagnosis of any kind. Without this ability, chiropractors would be entirely dependent upon the referral of a physician. In November 2006, a judge ruled that both of these procedures were outside the scope of practice for chiropractors, and chiropractors should not be allowed to diagnose subluxations or diagnose conditions beyond the spine and musculoskeletal system for the purpose of referring patients. The Texas Board of Chiropractors and The Texas Chiropractic Association, who joined the lawsuit, appealed.

In 2011, the Court of Appeals of Texas reviewed the case and found in favor of the Texas Board of Chiropractors in that chiropractors are permitted to diagnose subluxations of the spine or musculoskeletal system and outlined examples of what is in that scope of practice (Edwards, 2013). Many chiropractors hailed the 2011 case as a victory for the profession, particularly when the Supreme Court refused to hear the case on appeal (*Texas Board of Chiropractic Examiners v. Texas Medical Association*, Court of Appeals of Texas, Third District).

At the same time however, the Court of Appeals remanded the case back to the trial court for a full trial on its merits. TMA was successful in its bid to prohibit chiropractors from performing EMG treatments as well as spinal manipulations on patients under anesthesia (see Texas Medical Association, 2013).

The TMA then filed another lawsuit against the Board for its rule allowing chiropractors with special training to perform instrument assisted Vestibular Ocular Nystagmus Testing (VONT), which is designed to diagnose symptoms such as dizziness and an inability of patients to focus their vision after moving their head or neck.

In 2016 the TMA amended its lawsuit against the chiropractic Board to expand its attack on the diagnosis issue. The case is currently under appeal, but it is clear that the TMA has serious issues with chiropractors' scope of practice and their competency. The outcome of this case, if decided in favor of TMA, could have a significant deleterious impact on chiropractors across the country.

INTERNAL STRIFE WITHIN THE PROFESSION

As if the external threats to chiropractic were not enough, where many chiropractors feel as though the medical profession continues to discriminate against them, while health care reform hampers their ability to operate, there are internal challenges within the profession that serve to divide chiropractors and create a climate of mistrust. Some chiropractors, for example, feel that doctors are threatened by chiropractic medicine or they fear the loss of revenue if they refer patients to chiropractors.

As Mike points out,

> Doctors won't refer patients to us because they know chiropractic works, they're not stupid. But they don't refer them to us because they are worried that we will take that patient from them and they don't want to lose the money that patient brings to the office.

Another chiropractor, Vinnie, pointed out the following:

> I have talked to orthopedic doctors before and they admit that they can't send us patients because they need to work and can't afford to lose patients. I remember one guy when I was up in Delaware, I'll never forget this, I was working with another guy. And we decided to tag team the marketing of it all. And we went to the biggest MD in the area, brought lunch. Did a one-hour lunch for him and his staff, PAs, everything. The staff goes back to work, he stays with us for a

> minute or two before we go, and I go, "What did you think?" He says, "It was great! Great presentation, very informative for my staff. I appreciate it." And he said, "But if I send you my patients and I can't write my scripts, I'll be out of business." That's what he said to me. So it's not that they don't know, or don't know if it can be beneficial, it's that it's you or me.
>
> Here's another example. I had a satellite office in Delaware. And I worked out of an MD office. I met the guy playing golf and he said "Hey you can lease some space from me if you want." So I'm in there, and it was pretty archaic the way he had me do it, I mean like rolling in a cart, he was an asshole, but I'm working, I'm like six, seven months into this thing, and all of a sudden I get a call the doc wants to see you. I'm like okay, so I show up and he says, "This isn't going to work out." And I'm like "What do you mean?" He goes, "My patients are saying they're getting better and they don't want to take this," whatever he was prescribing and I was like "Wait a minute, I thought this was a tag team this was a collaboration for the patients and their health." He cut me loose that day.

This sense of persecution is a prevalent theme in the data—where chiropractors believe that doctors simply do not refer patients to them.

Kat points to a problem that an orthopedic surgeon mentioned in a previous chapter—the concern about referring a patient to a chiropractor because they do not know what type of treatments a patient might receive. Not only are doctors worried about this issue, chiropractors themselves have a similar concern. She says the following:

> To me, it's difficult to refer people to other chiropractors, because I don't know if they're going to get ultrasound or EMS (electric muscle stimulation) and then . . . some kind of traction. . . . I just don't know what's going to happen. I wish I just had a way to tell people, this person is just going to adjust you and that's what you need, so we can narrow down what's going on. . . . And I think it's hard for people to know, and I don't think people know what chiropractic is because when they go to a chiropractor, they get adjusted and a million other things done to them too . . . and that's what it is, it is just manipulation of joints.

Other chiropractors talk extensively about the devious practices of other chiropractors. As Clyde offers his experiences with the profession, one begins to get a sense of desperation or self-preservation some chiropractors feel in running practice, where ethics play a secondary role in how they operate. He says the following:

> Well, I used to be really involved in the profession. I was a member of the state association, went to the national conferences, got involved in all sorts of ways. But over time, I just had too many bad experiences. The state association doesn't seem interested in the real issues and is afraid to do anything

to anyone—and there aren't that many members to begin with. I also had a lot of bad experiences with chiropractors and other providers. People would come work for me and then leave because another chiropractor hired them at a better salary or easier workload and they would convince my patients to go with them. The chiropractor should have put a stop to that immediately, but everyone is trying to make money, so they turn a blind eye to it. Or if I came up with something new or a good way to bring patients to my practice, these guys would steal my idea and then use it—I mean I know we are all basically in competition with each other, especially here with so many chiropractors, but stealing patients, ideas and marketing suggestions? Are we that desperate? So once I realized the state association wasn't going to do anything and once I realized I couldn't trust my colleagues, I basically just stopped communicating with everyone. I hire a part-time guy now and then when I have to be out of town, but even he complains and wants more than he's worth. . . . Only a few of my patients will be seen by him-they just wait until I get back to be treated. So what am I paying him for? And then he complains that he doesn't get paid enough? It's a very isolating profession. I can't trust anybody to do the right thing.

As Doug points out:

There are problems with people in the profession making it hard for those of us who want to live ethically and gain some respect from the medical community. I mean we are really living hand to mouth. The only way we make any money is to get patients who have a good experience with us to refer us to someone they know. But that means you have to have patients to begin with and that's not always easy to do. I've been in the business for ten years now and I can tell you there are some real shady characters out there. Guys who will scare patients by saying that they have to be treated or they're going to die or have major health problems in the next six months. It's crazy. But some of these guys are smooth and can convince people that they need all this extra stuff the patient doesn't need.

Josh points out the following:

I don't share information with other chiropractors about anything. I don't give them tips on what types of advertising works for me, I don't talk specifics about any supplemental treatments I might do, I don't share anything and I only talk in terms of generalities when I go to meetings or meet other chiropractors. [Why?] Because you never know if someone is going to use that information to their advantage. Let's be honest, we are colleagues but we are all in competition with each other. So why would I give my competitor an edge voluntarily? I don't owe them anything and they will be the first ones to steal a patient if they get the chance. We are all struggling here and every patient counts. So you just can't be open and honest with people.

While there have undoubtedly been physicians who engage in unethical practices and while some may poach patients from another provider or take patients with them as they move to another practice or group, the problem appears to be more widespread in the chiropractic profession—most of the chiropractors who participated in this study either experienced something firsthand or knew of colleagues who had been victimized by chiropractors in a variety of ways.

Perhaps this is due to the economic challenges many chiropractors face, where there can be a need for some providers to maximize revenue for each patient. Not all chiropractors have to worry about this, as some practices are large and revenues are strong. During the interviews I consistently noted comments made by providers who indicated that most were struggling financially and their patient pool was dwindling. Many chiropractors also made comments about colleagues who had closed their practices or were on the verge of bankruptcy.

These factors perpetuate the atmosphere of mistrust, suspicion of other chiropractors, and an unwillingness to share information, insight, or successful techniques. It also leads some providers to engaging in questionable business practices, including diversification into areas that are questionable as well as engaging in questionable billing practices to insurance companies.

DISCUSSION

The lack of a unified voice within the profession poses a host of challenges for chiropractors, even those who profess disdain for some of their colleagues' unscrupulous tactics and strategies. Virtually every chiropractor interviewed for this project professed a strong opinion about the state of affairs in the profession and cited their colleagues as one of the strongest threats to the viability of the profession in the future. All seem to recognize that the autonomy so important to being a chiropractor has as a consequence an inability to agree on the most important issues within the profession.

Most of the chiropractors in the study also lament about what lies ahead for the profession because they do not believe that any progress toward a unified and collective voice will occur. So sharp are the divisions that these providers believe there is an inevitable shadow cast on the profession, one from which it may not recover. Kathleen says the following:

> But when you were talking about the main issue in chiropractic? I think it's chiropractors. It's the infighting and the lack of unification that's the biggest threat to the profession. I mean we can't agree on scope of practice. You have people from Life and Sherman that are just about adjusting and subluxation and we can

cure everything with adjustments, and we have people from National who are like "I want my chiropractor doing gynecological exams and cardiology exams on patients." I mean both are a little ridiculous. . . . And when you are that far to the extreme, you aren't going to get anywhere close to the middle. I think one of three things is going to happen with chiropractic. It's either going to die, and manual therapy is going to go to physical therapists and osteopaths, or we're going to get our shit together and figure out what our scope of practice is going to be and go that way, or we're going to lose our status as providers and just be technicians. . . . That's what I think. [Will that be difficult because a lot of MD's aren't going to want to refer?] Exactly. So two of those scenarios, chiropractic doesn't exist anymore.

Some chiropractors and those involved in the training of the next generation of providers are a bit optimistic about the future. These tend to be the Reformers, who have a sense that things have to be different in order for the profession to survive. But with that survival comes some very pragmatic steps and admissions that the chiropractic profession has not been willing to provide. John, a dean at one of the chiropractic colleges, had this to say:

The war that's going on is a political one not an academic one. What we have to do, the ACA is going through some transformations themselves. I know they changed their administrative structure, but they see it now if we are going to get anywhere, we are going to have to present ourselves in a more unified way. The International Chiropractic Association is cult-like and hopefully is on its way down and the ACA is on its way up. The other part of that is the profession statewide has got to have the balls to come down on unethical or unprofessional practices. I believe there is a lot of acceptance and turn a blind eye to a lot of things. You know when I was at Northwestern, we had a medical doctor that was on our board, a radiologist. And myself and another chiropractor were talking to him about some of this silliness, and he said, he was blunt, from his perspective as an elderly MD, he saw it differently. He said, "why do you put up with it? We wouldn't put up with that crap in the medical profession."

And he's right. And I think part of the reason we put up with it is that it's our dirty little secret that we don't want to expose it as a house of cards, but sooner or later the profession has to come down hard on the unethical elements and prove to the public that it really can police itself properly. And this coupled with better qualified graduates who don't practice by pseudo-science, all these things take place slowly, but if we can do it quick enough to establish trust, then maybe we can become the podiatrists of the spine, which is what we need to do right now. And it's tragic, but here's the sad thing, when I went to school we just called it chiropractic, if you're in . . . pick a country, and you have a toothache, you'll probably get the same type of treatment as you would if you were in New Jersey. But in chiropractic in one city, you could go to twenty different chiropractors, some will do spinal manipulation, some will use the silly

> little activator gun, some would use the soft tissue technique with the stainless steel instruments that look like butter knives on your back or neck for heaven's sake, some don't do anything and some will use energy techniques, some will do rehab, some will do massage, some will do trigger point, it's bizarre. You got a hundred different approaches to the same thing, and it's embarrassing. I don't know to what extent there is some element of uniformity that is emerging, but some of these practices are still encouraged by schools. I mean, activators are just crazy, it's bizarre. It's a popular form or technique, and I don't know why, and frankly if I was an insurance company I wouldn't pay for that.
>
> [I have heard that depending on the techniques you perform, you get beat up, and the activator is a less intense adjustment, but it helps ease the stress on the provider.]
>
> You are bang on with that. . . . And the other thing is that hasn't been mentioned is whether it's clinically effective. They tout the research on it, but the research isn't clinical effectiveness, the research is how many people feel better. And then these new grads wonder why aren't we respected. I'm hoping we're on the right track on some issues. And some of the schools are jumping on to the evidence-based model than they have in the past, so we have to feel good about where we are headed.

In fact, many of the more thoughtful members of the profession, those who are either engaging in research or are writing about important issues in the profession, agree as well. A recent issue of the *Journal of Chiropractic Humanities* focused on the theme of professional identity. Many of the articles lamented the lack of identity in the profession and its need to establish one, but all fell short of calling for the creation of a mechanism or entity to require minimum standards of accountability. Such measures are part and parcel to the creation of a professional identity, as evidenced in other professions.

While there are many specialty areas in medicine, in law, in engineering, and even in academia, all operate on the basis of some type of limits in terms of what is allowable, ethical, and appropriate. This has not happened in chiropractic medicine and is a serious obstacle to its viability in the future. This is particularly true given that most people do not understand what chiropractors do, are fearful of their treatment, and/or suspect ulterior motives in their practices. This is not to say that all chiropractors have to believe and act the same way, but it does mean that unless there are reasonable limits placed on providers, they will continue to engage in a wide range of activities which will cause confusion and suspicion of chiropractors and of the profession in general.

With regard to the discussion of vertebral subluxations, it seems as though this idea was originally created along with a terminology and range of treatments to keep chiropractors out of jail for practicing without a license. Somewhere along the way, perhaps through repetition, it was given some level of credibility, particularly when the issues of licensure and insurance reimbursement became relevant to the discussion. While there are many chiropractors who are gaining some distance from the term and the idea, preferring the use of other terms to describe what may be happening when patients are injured, because so much of the profession's identity and purpose is tied to the subluxation, it is difficult to imagine chiropractic medicine without that phrase being part of the narrative, despite the stigma associated with it.

More pragmatically, some observers have noted that the reason for the controversy is not because there is a belief that subluxations actually exist, but eliminating it from the discussions of chiropractic medicine would likely render the profession irrelevant and relegate it to a minor role in medicine, such as pain management. As many chiropractors have pointed out in our discussions, if they are not careful, the profession will be "eaten" by medicine. Others point out that many chiropractors are "selling out" their ideology by trying to act like physicians.

For whatever the reasons, this fear of becoming irrelevant is an important motivator, and because so many chiropractors have hung their proverbial hats on the subluxation as a defining feature of what they do—it will be difficult if not impossible to distinguish chiropractors from physical therapists, osteopaths, or even massage therapists since they also perform a number of common techniques. As an illustration, one chiropractor sharply rebuked me in an interview when I mentioned that some patients have said they felt like they were "in alignment" after receiving a massage. He said, "No! No! No! Massage therapy isn't the same thing as a chiropractic adjustment. They are totally different!" The intensity of this defensive response was striking and noteworthy.

At the same time, however, if chiropractic is not about actually adjusting the spine or moving bones, is it not reasonable to question the defining characteristic of chiropractic medicine, especially if others already perform these treatments? No wonder the guy got so defensive. It seems, then, that the vertebral subluxation will likely remain a part of the discussion because, despite evidence to the contrary, it is difficult to admit mistakes of the past. Some chiropractors still cling to the dogma that suggests there is a spiritual element to chiropractic medicine, which further complicates the issue.

While criticisms of chiropractic medicine abound, it seems reasonable to conclude that pain is an indicator that something is going on in the joint or the muscles surrounding it—pain and restricted mobility are important diagnostic variables. Given what the evidence shows, that the original understanding about the subluxation cannot definitively be proven, is chiropractic treatment simply a fabrication of the past? It is fair to conclude that something is going on with that painful area and to suggest that chiropractic treatment does something for some people to relieve that pain and restore mobility to the joint—whether chiropractic is unique in that treatment or whether other treatments are just as effective (including doing nothing) is a topic for another discussion.

The conclusion in a recent article by the *Journal of the American Medical Association*, one that so many chiropractors point to for validation, suggests that the weight of the evidence is that spinal manipulation is one type of treatment that appears to have a mildly positive effect.

With regard to understanding how chiropractors see themselves and how they are seen by others, sociologically perhaps the best concept or theory that provides a bit of understanding of this process is a theory developed by Charles Horton Cooley called the *Looking Glass Self Theory*. In his 1902 book, *Human Nature and the Social Order*, Cooley outlined his idea of the Looking Glass Self theory. He says the following: a self-idea of this sort seems to have three principle elements:

1. The imagination of our appearance to the other person.
2. The imagination of his judgment of that appearance.
3. Some sort of self-feeling such as pride or mortification.

In other words, Cooley says we imagine how other people see us and we also imagine how they evaluate our "presentation of self" or how we present ourselves in the course of our interactions with others. As we consider those imagined evaluations others make about us, we draw conclusions and generate real emotions and feelings, not only about how we acted in those specific situations also about our identity.

The key component to all of this, however, are those imagined evaluations. We are not very adept at interpreting those imagined evaluations, where we usually think people see us in the worse possible light. Cooley reminds us that such assessments can easily lead to erroneous understanding of ourselves as well as causing us to think, believe, and act very differently than we might otherwise if those evaluations were positive ones.

In the case of chiropractors, much of how they believe they are perceived in medicine is found in their understanding of how physicians and traditional medicine view them. Because this is generally negative, feelings of inferiority and persecution are seen in many of the comments offered in this study. Chiropractors also mentioned how they feel slighted as medical professionals and their inability to successfully operate a practice is based on the idea that medical doctors will not refer patients to them. But these perceptions are not necessarily based in objective facts. Most physicians interviewed for this study may not agree with chiropractic care as a legitimate form of treatment, but that is very different from a dislike of chiropractors. Thus, the emotions, attitudes, beliefs, and conclusions described by chiropractors are based on their imagined evaluations or misinterpretations of interactions with others.

Thus, the tendency for chiropractors to describe themselves as members of a persecuted at the hands of the medical community comes not from any actual effort by physicians, but by the perceptions of chiropractors that traditional medicine is against them. Consequently, chiropractors think less of themselves and of their own profession. This is the essence of the looking glass theory—who we are and what we think of ourselves is a product of our interactions with others and our understanding (correctly or incorrectly) of how they see us.

Finally, with regard to the internal strife within the profession, virtually every chiropractor in this study pointed out that the inability to gain a consensus, to "get their act together" or to rid the profession of the quacks and the frauds, perpetually keeps chiropractic from legitimacy. Yet, no one in the profession seems willing to take the necessary steps to do what needs to be done. Instead, many chiropractors are content to lament the state of affairs, to offer story after story about how traditional medicine inappropriately mistreats chiropractors and to complain about the lack of success in terms of credibility and a strong professional identity. In reality, chiropractors have found themselves in a situation where, as Kathleen points out, they are "their own worst enemy."

In the next chapter we explore a recent development in chiropractic medicine, one that represents a challenge to the autonomy of chiropractors and their sense of independence. The Joint franchise has been derisively referred to as the "Walmart of Chiropractic" and has caused yet another layer of controversy within the profession. The issues surrounding this new model of treating patients will be explored in greater depth as it extends the discussion of the scope of practice, the philosophy of treatment, and the idea of maintenance therapy within the profession. Particularly since it threatens to change the business model used in chiropractic offices, the Joint provides yet another issue that creates questions about the profession's credibility.

REFERENCES

American Academy of Family Physicians. 2017. *Needle Electromyography*. Available at http://www.aafp.org/dam/AAFP/documents/advocacy/workforce/scope/ES-NeedleElectromyography-0605.pdf

Arnold, J. J. and Ehleringer, S. R. 2012. "Is Spinal Manipulation an Effective Treatment for Low Back Pain? Yes: Evidence Shows Benefit in Most Patients." *American Family Physician*, April 15th, 85(8): 756–758.

Bialosky, J. E., Bishop, Robinson, M. E. 2009. "Spinal Manipulative Therapy has an Immediate Effect on Thermal Pain Sensitivity in People with Low Back Pain: A Randomized Controlled Trial." *Physical Therapy* 89(12): 1292–1303.

Bronfort, G., Haas, M., and Evans, R. L. 2004. "Efficacy of Spinal Manipulation and Mobilization for Low Back Pain and Neck Pain: A Systematic Review and Best Evidence Synthesis." *Spine Journal* 4(3): 335–356.

Cherkin, D. C., Sherman, K. J., and Deyo, R. A. 2003. "A Review of the Evidence for the Effectiveness, Safety, and Cost of Acupuncture, Massage Therapy, and Spinal Manipulation for Back Pain." *Annals of Internal Medicine* 138(11): 898–906.

Cooley, C. H. 1902. *Human Nature and the Social Order*. New York: Scribner's and Sons, pp. 179–185.

Edwards, J. 2013. "Texas Medical Association Denied." *Dynamic Chiropractic*, 31(15), August 1st. Available at https://dynamicchiropractic.com/mpacms/dc/article.php?id=56584

Ernst, E. and Posadzki, P. 2011. "An Independent Review of NCCAM-funded Studies of Chiropractic." *Clinical Rheumatology* 30: 593–600.

Feise, R. J. 2001. "Reliability of Chiropractic Methods Commonly Used to Detect Maniputable Lesions in Patients with Chronic Low-Back Pain." *Journal of Manipulative Physiological Therapy* 24(2): 145–146.

Hall, H. 2014. "Top 10 Chiropractic Studies of 2013." *Science-Based Medicine*, January 21st. Available at https://sciencebasedmedicine.org/top-10-chiropractic-studies-of-2013/

Illinois Chiropractic Society. 2012. *Scope of Practice*. Available at http://www.ilchiro.org/news/128631/The-Chiropractic-Scope-in-Illinois.htm

Long, P. H. 2013. *Chiropractic Abuse: An Insider's Lament*. New York: American Council on Science and Health.

Morgan, L. 1998. "Innate Intelligence: Its Origins and Problems." *Journal of the Chiropractic Association* 42(1): 38.

Qaseem, A., Wilt, T. J., McClean, R. M., and Forciea, M. A. 2017. "Non-Invasive Treatment for Acute, Subacute, and Chronic Low Back Pain: A Clinical Practice Guideline from the American College of Physicians." *Annals of Internal Medicine* 166: 514–530. Available at https://www.ncbi.nlm.nih.gov/pubmed/28192789

State of South Carolina, Department of Labor, Licensing and Regulation. 2017. *Chiropractor's Scope of Practice*. Available at http://www.llr.state.sc.us/pol/chiropractors/index.asp?file=scope.htm

Texas Medical Association. 2016. "Court Sides with TMA in Final Ruling in Chiropractic Scope of Practice." November 1st. Available at https://www.texmed.org/Template.aspx?id=43704

U.S. Department of Health and Human Services, Office of Inspector General, 2016. *Hundreds of Millions in Medicare Payments for Chiropractic Services did not Comply with Medicare Requirements*. Available at https://oig.hhs.gov/oas/reports/region9/91402033.pdf

Chapter 5

The Joint and Discounted Chiropractic Care

As we saw in the last chapter, the issue of scope of practice is a thorny one and relates to many aspects of chiropractic medicine. Belief in the existence of vertebral subluxations, the need for maintenance therapy, long-standing disagreements within the profession, and a lack of trust among providers are generally related to the issue of scope of practice. This is true despite the fact that South Carolina has one of the more narrowly defined legal parameters surrounding a chiropractor's scope of practice. Another theme that drives much of the discussion of chiropractic medicine is this notion of autonomy.

The fiercely independent ideas held by many chiropractors is one of the profession's defining features, but the flip side to that autonomy is an inability or unwillingness to agree on central issues in the profession, a lack of a unified collective voice, and, perhaps most importantly, an unwillingness to hold colleagues accountable who push the boundaries of acceptable behavior. Unlike other professions, as Doug mentioned in one of our conversations, the public, and, to some extent, the medical community, can paint the behavior of the unscrupulous chiropractors and those who genuinely try to help patients with the same broad brush; the behavior of a select few puts all chiropractors under a negative spotlight. While this is obviously unreasonable, the profession has to bear some responsibility by its unwillingness to self-regulate and to cast out those chiropractors who engage in questionable or fraudulent practices.

Thus, while autonomy and independence have a host of influences in chiropractic medicine, I was curious to learn more about how chiropractors and those involved in chiropractic education felt about the development of the Joint. This is a franchise business that provides inexpensive adjustments to patients and its model contains a host of features not provided by traditional chiropractors. The Joint's methods are a bit unusual and attempts to appeal to that segment of the population that may not have experienced chiropractic treatment. I spent time with franchise owners, chiropractors who work as employees of the Joint, and asked the chiropractors, deans, and provosts who participated in the study about its impact on the profession.

THE JOINT

In 1999, a chiropractor, who was likely involved in the controversial subject of maintenance care for chiropractic patients, began to imagine how he could transform chiropractic medicine by making treatments more convenient and affordable. In 2010, the Joint was founded with eight franchised clinics. Since then, according to their website, the company has expanded nationwide into 370 clinics, offering more than four million spinal adjustments per year (The Joint.com).

Its mission is "to improve the quality of life through routine and affordable chiropractic care." The idea, then, is to increase awareness of chiropractic treatment and its value to the average person who may not understand what chiropractors do. Another goal is to make treatments easy, convenient, and affordable. The CEO of the Joint, Peter Holt, points out that "for years, chiropractic was dismissed as unscientific by the traditional medical industry and to some extent, a large percentage of the American population" (The Joint.com).

The company accomplishes this through the use of maintenance plans and treatment packages that offer a wide range of options and fees, similar to a gym membership, where patients receive a greater discount for the larger package they purchase. The plans are not covered by insurance, which is said to eliminate the administrative headaches of claims, reimbursements, and copays. Patients simply sign up for a plan and can visit any clinic anywhere in the country up to four times per month. The average cost for a plan is $59 per month. The Joint has locations all over the United States with expanded hours of operation, usually 10 am to 7 pm, and offices are open on Saturdays and Sundays, a rarity in the chiropractic profession, and no appointments are needed. Patients can come whenever it is convenient for them.

Data on the Success of the Joint

According to its Franchise Disclosure Document, the projected growth of Joint franchises was significant in 2016 and while it currently has 370 clinics, the goal is to open over 1,700 locations across the country. The average gross sale of all clinics was $320,765, which is $60,000 more than what traditional chiropractic clinics reported that year. The Joint also sees more patients than most chiropractors, with an average of 257 patients per week, compared to approximately 100 for traditional clinics (The Joint.com).

In a traditional chiropractic office, with the use of insurance and copays, the average cost to a patient is approximately $40 and the rest is billed to the insurance company. In contrast, the average cost per visit for a patient at the Joint is $23 to $26. No insurance is used and there are no administrative costs connected to the visit (Why the Joint is an Attractive Business Model, 2017). Officials at the Joint believe this model has rejuvenated the chiropractic profession which, they contend, was in decline. Part of the reason had to do with decreased reimbursements by third-party insurance carriers.

A review of the website includes a claim that chiropractors are the highest rated health care practitioners for low back pain treatments, above physical therapists, specialist physicians/MDs, and primary care physicians. This is according to the National Center for Complementary and Integrative Health. The article cites a *Consumer Reports* article, which offers many facts about chiropractic treatments, including a 2007 National Health Interview Survey, which found that adults in the United States spent nearly $12 billion in out-of-pocket expenses on visits to complementary health practitioners, nearly $4 billion of which was spent on chiropractic or osteopathic manipulations.

Other data cited on the Joint website points out that some research indicates that spinal manipulation appears to benefit some people and may also be helpful for headaches, neck pain, extremity joint conditions, and whiplash associated disorders. As is pointed out, a 2010 review of evidence on manual therapies concluded that the spinal manipulation may be helpful for some conditions, such as migraine headaches, but is not helpful for ailments such as asthma, hypertension, and menstrual pain. Inconclusive evidence has been found to deal with fibromyalgia, mid-back pain, sciatica, and temporomandibular joint disorders—or jaw problems.

However, while this evidence appears to promote the use of chiropractic treatments, it is subject to interpretation and does not definitively show that chiropractic medicine definitively helps. As discussed in the previous chapter, the research on chiropractic care seems to suggest that treatments may help, but it does not appear that they are any better than other traditional remedies. While it may make some sense that chiropractors know more about back problems than primary care physicians and perhaps some other medical specialists, it is not clear that what they actually do is demonstrably better than any other remedy that is available and some of the conclusions on the Joint's website suffer from some inaccuracies.

For instance, in referencing the data point that chiropractors are the highest rated practitioners for back and neck pain, the website cites a *Consumer Reports* study. In 2012, *Consumer Reports* conducted a survey of over 45,000 users of that magazine about alternative medicine uses and found that acupuncture, chiropractic treatment, and massage therapy were far less helpful than prescription medicine for most of the conditions. As the article states,

> Despite the hoopla over alternative treatments, when we asked respondents how well the therapies they used worked for 12 common health problems, results showed that they were usually deemed far less helpful than prescription medicine for most of the conditions. (consumerrreports.org)

The article also points out, correctly, that this survey, despite its size, is not representative of the entire population. They say the following:

> Respondents based their opinions on personal experience so the results can't be compared with scientific clinical trials. And our results do not take into account the power of the placebo effect, the tendency of people to find even simulated or sham interventions helpful. (consumerreports.org)

Interestingly, this article makes no mention of chiropractors as the highest rated provider for low back pain, despite the fact that it is used as the source for that claim. Perhaps this was an oversight and perhaps a bit of image enhancement is occurring, where interpretations of selected data allow the Joint to engage in a bit of impression management (Goffman, 1969), particularly with people who know little or nothing about chiropractic treatments.

The fact that the profession generates $14 billion revenue each year should make one wonder about why so many chiropractors complain about not being more successful. Then again, the Bureau of Labor Statistics states that in 2016, the average salary for a chiropractor was $81,210 with a median salary of $67,520 (Bureau of Labor Statistics, 2016). If chiropractors are seen as mid-level providers, as indicated by their salaries, how does one account for $14 billion in revenue? As Jerry, a franchise owner, points out, not all data can be considered reliable and trustworthy.

Many of the franchise owners are chiropractors, who benefit from the brand, the convenient locations, and the cash-only business model. Many chiropractors point out that the administrative costs associated with reimbursement from insurance companies, particularly since they only get a fraction of their normal fees, make a cash model much more efficient and profitable.

Parenthetically, many chiropractors in the study lamented about insurance reimbursements but were fearful of converting to a cash model since so many of their patients use insurance coverage to pay for treatment. The Joint appears to embrace the cash model from the outset and presents it to patients as a form of convenience. Most patients do not really feel the effects of the reimbursement process by insurance companies, except when the policy reaches its limit in terms of coverage. Most of the administrative challenges offered by chiropractors occur between the provider and the insurance company, that is, until the provider informs the patient of the lack of coverage and they are then required to pay cash for treatment.

In addition to chiropractors who purchase franchises from the Joint, many franchise owners are also entrepreneurs, who see the value in the low buy-in costs, quick turnaround, and simplicity of the business model. With startup costs less than $400,000 and the simplicity of the operational model, with minimal staff and the absence of expensive equipment or accessories, business-minded people can quickly recoup their initial investment. Thus, in many ways, the Joint represents what appears to be a successful business model in the chiropractic profession, one that is attracting new patients to treatment (the website claims that the average number of new patients per month across all clinics in 2016 was approximately 19) and seems to have solved several of the most persistent problems in the profession.

THE CHIROPRACTIC COMMUNITY'S RESPONSE

Based on the responses from those interviewed for this study, the Joint evokes a level of hostility that is perhaps greater than any other topic. There were a few providers in the study who actually worked for the Joint on a part-time basis, so they had some level of understanding of the operation and the philosophy of the Joint that others did not, but the response was almost unanimous: they believe the Joint represents a threat to the industry and the profession because it is unsafe, dangerous, and risky to patients.[1] As one of the deans of a chiropractic college stated, he thinks the Joint disparages the profession more so than chiropractors who engage in dubious treatments. He says the following:

> We have them in our state. I'm totally 100% against that because before you do any adjusting you have to do a really good history a really good exam, a good diagnosis and treatment plan . . . and they don't do that. I was on a panel with the ACA about this and it was a resolution that you can't provide treatment with a proper diagnosis and you can't provide a proper diagnosis without a history and exam. So they are really hurting the profession, because they are so substandard compared to what's being taught and what's being expected, but they haven't been tried yet. At some point in time, someone will get hurt and there'll be a trial, but the problem is that once that happens, like in most circumstances, when they go down, it will be an indictment of the whole profession.

Safety Concerns

The comments and criticisms of the Joint offered by chiropractors in this study focused heavily on the safety of patients. Many of the providers who participated in the study are strong proponents of the vertebral subluxation, itself a rather controversial subject, who generally dismiss criticisms of chiropractic adjustments as unsafe by physicians and others. These same providers claim that the Joint and its employees pose a risk of injury to patients. This occurs despite the fact that the Joint hires only licensed chiropractors who graduated from some of the same accredited institutions from which they are alumni. Jimmy, a chiropractor in the study, says the following:

> How can they provide quality care? There's no X-ray, there is no real diagnosis of a problem other than what the patient tells them is wrong. People come in, lay down, get adjusted and that's it? And we call this quality chiropractic care? Someone is going to get hurt. I assume they have licensed chiropractors working for them or are they chiropractic assistants? [my understanding is that they are licensed chiropractors.] Well, then they are probably substandard chiropractors because I can't imagine anyone being willing to adjust a patient without an X-ray and thorough evaluation.

My own observations of this particular chiropractor showed that most of the patients who came into Jimmy's office routinely received the same adjustment every time and there was no follow-up or routine x-rays beyond the initial consultation. Typically, the provider would palpate the patient, ask them how they were feeling, and focus on the area that the patient said was troubling to them. My observations of providers at the Joint did the same thing. One particular chiropractor was very critical of the Joint because its providers were not identifying subluxations, which, he says, is critical to treating a patient. John says the following:

> How can they operate safely and effectively? They can't! You mean to tell me that a chiropractor working at the Joint is going to be able to palpate a patient and identify a subluxation and correct it all without an X-ray and by doing so with a quick conversation with a patient? I can't believe they let these guys get away with that kind of nonsense.
>
> Everyone knows that you need an X-ray to identify a subluxation. [Do you take X-rays of patients every time they come into your office?] No, but I have a patient history to know where to look. If a patient typically has mid-back problems, then I know to focus on that area unless he tells me that his neck or upper back are bothering him. [So if a patient has a subluxation in one area of the back that means he or she is likely to always have them there? Is that why you focus on that part of the spine and not do an X-ray?] Well, you can't do regular X-rays, that's bad for the patient to be exposed to that much radiation. But yes, I generally tend to concentrate on where the problem was before, but that can only come with a detailed history of the patient.

Notice the inconsistency in this chiropractor's comments. He has the ability to identify a subluxation by palpating the patient and he knows it is there because he has seen it on an X-ray. This is true despite the controversy surrounding the actual presence of subluxations and the ability of chiropractors to accurately and consistently identify them, either on an X-ray or by examining a patient (Magner and Barrett, 1995; Long, 2012). He is critical of providers at the Joint for doing the very things he does in his everyday practice. Thus, the issue is not really a safety concern for the patient. Likely it is the fact that the Joint represents competition for patients at a discounted price. This is conjecture of course, but it seems hard to defend an argument against a colleague who uses the same diagnostic techniques on patients, but simply charges less for the service.

Undercutting the Market

Other chiropractors complain about the low cost treatment, sometimes referring to the Joint as the Walmart or McDonald's of chiropractic medicine. As Mike says, this puts a lot of pressure on current providers to justify their costs for services, which they feel is already below market value. He says the following:

> I already charge what I think is a really low price for my services. [How much is it to receive treatment, assuming the patient doesn't have insurance?] I charge $50 per visit, which I think is cheaper than most chiropractors in the area. But how can I compete with the Joint, when they charge $29 per visit and no appointments are needed? How do I compete with a maintenance plan that, at $59 per month, amounts to less than $20 per office visit if they come four times a month? With the amount of time I spend on billing issues with insurance companies and Medicare, I can't afford to stay in business if I charged that much. But I think the patient isn't aware of the fact that they are getting substandard care. [How is what you provide different from what they get at the Joint?] Well, to begin with, I spend a lot of time trying to get to know my patients and to learn about their families and their hobbies and what their health goals are—then I try to counsel them on how to achieve those goals. So I provide a service that is much more comprehensive than this discounted, "in and out" type of treatment offered by the Joint, where you never know which doctor is going to be there and if he even remembers your name.

This provider believes that he offers a value-added service to his patients by virtue of his concern for their well-being, the time he spends getting to know them, and learning more about how they want to remain active. This, he says, cannot be calculated in terms of a cost per visit, but the Joint is undercutting all chiropractors by advertising a bargain basement price. This, he says, undermines the holistic approach chiropractors take in treating patients. As he points out, "there is much, much, more to chiropractic treatment than simply getting an adjustment."

Forcing Chiropractors to Work Harder

Mike's observations may have some merit in that the Joint's presence in the market requires chiropractors in private practice to offer additional explanation to their patients about the added value of what they are receiving that Joint employees do not provide. It has also put pressure on providers to consider expanding their current operational protocols. As Kat points out, some chiropractors complain that they now have to consider offering better service to their patients, something that chiropractors often point to as a distinguishing feature between their treatments and conventional medicine. She says the following:

> So many people say "I don't want to give up my lunch break on a Tuesday or give up my Saturday." And I'm like "Well, then get a regular job where you can sit at a desk and clock out at five o'clock."

It is not uncommon to see chiropractic offices closed for lunch for two and a half hours during the days when it is open a full day and most chiropractic offices are not open every day. Many chiropractors have stated that they need this extended time to recover from the physical demands that result from treating patients. The upshot, of course, is that patients have a limited opportunity to schedule an appointment. With two-and-a-half hour lunch break as the norm, patients can schedule appointments or visit an office in the morning, typically from 9 am to about noon, and then again from 3 pm to 5 pm.

A typical office will have these hours about two days per week and a shortened schedule on the others days, perhaps only 9 am to 12 pm or 2 pm to 5 pm. Most are not open on weekends or later hours. Thus the window of opportunity to visit a chiropractor is predicated on their schedule, not the patient's needs. Thus, while a commitment to the patient's needs is something that virtually every chiropractor extols as a unique aspect to chiropractic medicine, often in response to a criticism of traditional medicine's insensitivity to patients, it appears that for many chiropractors, the normal hours of operation are incongruent with when patients can show up for treatment. Perhaps this is one reason why so many chiropractors in the study have struggled financially—they are not open as often or as long as when patients need their services. As one chiropractor pointed out, "These guys at the Joint are eating my lunch and there's nothing I can do about it. I don't know what I'm going to do, but I can't keep losing patients and expect to stay in business much longer."

In contrast, the Joint is open on Saturdays and has extended hours so that patients who end their workday at 5 pm can make it to a location and receive treatment after work. The hours of operation of several franchises that I observed were Monday through Friday 10 am to 7 pm and Saturdays from 10 am to 4 pm. And because no appointments are required, patients can simply show up when it is convenient for them.

Philosophical Differences

Some chiropractors point to the idea of maintenance therapy as the primary tool used by the Joint. This is a highly debatable issue and the controversy surrounding it extends to the business model used by the Joint. As Jake, a chiropractor, pointed out,

> So instead they tell you that you need regular maintenance as part of a wellness program that keeps you active and healthy. Well, who wouldn't consider that as an option when it's presented that way? What they aren't telling you, and what a lot of my colleagues who do that too, aren't telling you, is that you don't need that to remain healthy. What ever happened to the balanced approach to life? Everything is extremes and even chiropractic, which is supposed to know better and to be all about symmetry and balance, doesn't practice what they preach. Why? Because it isn't about the patient, it's about money. And many chiropractors have sold out just like doctors and pharmaceutical companies and insurance companies and everyone else. We are all a bunch of used car salesmen at the end of the day because we are more concerned with getting paid than with helping people.

Without a regular maintenance plan, like a gym membership, franchises like the Joint could not likely survive. The model is predicated on a volume of patients rather than maximizing the amount charged to each one. But what if the idea of maintenance therapy is shown to be unnecessary? As one dean of a chiropractic college points out, "It does not involve hurting people, as some of the research shows that prophylactic spinal manipulation does not injure patients, but it does nothing to improve their health. But at $59 per month with no end in sight, is this something that most patients would do if they knew it had no benefit?" As Josh, a provider, points out,

> The whole business model falls apart if they can't get a high volume of patients coming in the door. It ISN'T like a gym membership, where you need to exercise three times a week to stay healthy. You DON'T need to go to a chiropractor once a week to stay in alignment. I know I'm going to catch hell for this from my colleagues, who think that is the way the business operates, but that maintenance therapy stuff is for YOU, not for the patient. Prove to me that maintenance therapy has any scientific value—that's why insurance companies won't pay for it—and I think it is dishonest of providers, including the Joint, for selling it as a part of a wellness program.

> It doesn't do anything—now, if you need an adjustment and you want the flexibility of going whenever you want, that's one thing. That's up to you as a patient—you are paying a price for that convenience, but that is your choice. But that's not how they sell it to people.

Some of the chiropractors interviewed for this study, who are typically early in their careers and have not yet made the decision to open their own practice, also worked at the Joint part-time to make ends meet. Their observations about the operation of the Joint focus more on the details and challenges of being an employee. As Kat points out,

> It's tough. You are seeing 50 to 80 patients a day. You have to stay in shape or you're going to get hurt. And you're tired by the end of the day. . . . The last adjustment of the day isn't going to be as good as my first fifteen. It's two doctors working long shifts with no lunch breaks. So the Joint needs to do something about lunch breaks and half shifts instead of full shifts . . . or not just having two doctors at the clinics all the time. I think they'll work out the bugs. . . . Obviously franchisees are looking for money, so more than two doctors increase their overhead. . . . But there are benefits to working there. I don't have to worry about getting more patients, billing issues, marketing stuff, when I leave, I'm done. The hours are long and the pay isn't that great, but there is also freedom in just being an employee.

Other chiropractors have become employees of the Joint because they have retired from private practice and the Joint represents a way to remain active but they are relieved of the burdens of operating a business. Other chiropractors have found that they need to moonlight at the Joint while they operate a current practice because they simply cannot make ends meet on their own. Thus, the Joint serves many purposes for those in the chiropractic profession. Steve points to some of his experiences working at the Joint:

> Working there can be tough on you. . . . You have to take care of yourself. I've gotten hurt before . . . especially overuse injuries . . . that might be a byproduct of doing it after a while . . . that's why people switch to activator method after a while because it's so much easier on you. It doesn't have the same impact. . . . I don't see many chiropractors over 60. . . . It's very physically demanding. . . . there is something about the wear and tear on you . . . when you're the fulcrum you can't expect not to break down a bit.

Jack points to some of his experiences working at the Joint:

> I can give you a few minutes for that. When I first got out . . . when you first hear about it, the Joint sucks . . . the guy I work for now full-time as an Associate encouraged me to get a job at the Joint. Our goal at the Joint . . . it was either a

survey or census that about ten percent of people in the U.S. use chiropractors . . . that means 90 percent aren't. And it's because they don't know what it is, or cost prohibitive, or it's hard to access. . . . You can't go out of town and find a guy. So the idea behind the Joint is to reach out and access new patients. There are so many other people out there to market to . . . and they get a lot of flak because of the membership . . . . And ideally you'd want to get adjusted once a week so they have a program four adjustments in a month for a reasonable fee and you subscribe for a year. . . . Some people will sign this contract and then decide they don't want to do it, but it's a contract and they're locked into it.

Some people get pretty pissed about that when they can't get out of the contract, but the idea is to make it as accessible as possible to people who don't know about chiropractic and get them in and under consistent care. And then also to have a place that people are familiar with . . . . So you go to the Joint here and go out to California and throw your back out, you're like "where do I go? I bet there's a Joint around here." And so it has a bad rep depending on where you go, and they do have a lot of headway to make in terms of the workload on the staff, because it's a heavy workload if you're not used to it. . . . I don't think it's that bad . . . see they have long hours and you'll go in from 10–7. So long days, but most people don't work that as their full-time job. They do it hourly . . . and that's the other thing that people don't like, it's like I saw 25 patients today and got paid the same as when I saw zero patients. And I'm like yeah, but you still got paid when you saw zero patients. That's the balance.

[Depending on where you go, is there continuity of care?]

If it's run well, then you will have two or three doctors that come in on a schedule and you know when to come in to see who you like.

[So is it the case that you get guys that are retired? It's steady work, no headaches of running a practice or people like you that are doing it as a supplement until they get to where they want with their own practice?]

I think one guy I know sold them his practice and when it opened as the Joint, he was like coming back part-time and he's ramped up his hours because he doesn't have to worry about any of the other garbage. It's a good deal.

[Is it physically taxing on you?]

Yes. That's part of it for sure. You get beat up with that volume of patients. . . . You have to take care of yourself. I've gotten hurt before. . . . especially overuse injuries . . . that might be a byproduct of doing it after a while . . . that's why people switch to activator method after a while because it's so much easier on you. It doesn't have the same impact. . . . It's very physically demanding. . . . There is something about the wear and tear on you.

Other chiropractors who are employees of the Joint express some philosophical issues with the operation, such as the decision to treat patients. Kathleen says the following:

There are people that come into the Joint that I refuse to treat without an X-ray because of some type of trauma. I had one girl, she was about ten or eleven

> years old, she was playing on the monkey bars in school, fell on her head and felt this electrical sensation go all through her body and into her arms. Her mother brought her in because her mom doesn't like doctors. . . . And I'm like "Look has she had an X-ray or MRI or anything?" . . . and I said "She needs to see her primary care or ER to make sure she's okay. . . . Because if she has even a hairline fracture in her neck and I adjust her neck she's going to be a quadrapalegic. . . . And you're going to be really pissed off at me." And the mom argued with me about it and I said, "I'm not going to do it." [So does the Joint primarily focus on routine cases or people who already see a chiropractor?]
>
> Their whole thing is like a wellness type of deal. So we do see some like personal injury cases, but I tend to refer out if they aren't going to get better, and some doctors don't, they are sold on the plan no matter what they do, they give them the same adjustment. So it really depends on the doctor you see there. And I think eventually the Joint will have some issues with lawsuits in the future. It's just a matter of time because you're seeing so many people. If each clinic is seeing 80 patients a day or even 50, eventually something is going to happen. And if you have a lot of docs coming in with different training . . . you can pick your doctor, or you prefer so and so . . . the customer can wait. . . . I don't know if all Joints do it that way, but that's how we do it . . . the more you have on the schedule.

During the course of my time with chiropractors, staff members, deans, and provosts of chiropractic colleges around the country, and anyone affiliated with the chiropractic profession, none had anything really positive to say about the Joint and what they represent to the profession. Those who work as employees of the Joint offer a bit more insight, likely the result of knowing more of the facts and details about how the model operates, but aside from polite refrains from criticizing an employer or colleague, from the perspective of the chiropractic community, the Joint represents yet another attack on the profession. As Mike points out, "It's another example of the profession getting battered by someone. If it isn't doctors being unwilling to work with us, or insurance companies cutting our reimbursements, Medicare auditing the heck out of us, or other chiropractors don't steal patients and good employees, now we have to deal with this crap too? I mean, really? How much of this stuff are we expected to take?"

Mike's comments resonate with other chiropractors, who tend to feel as though they are not treated fairly in the profession or given a legitimate chance to earn a living. Granted, Mike's practice has about thirty patients a week at this point, so he may be feeling the effects of a declining practice and an uncertain future. Thus, his comments may be a reflection of the frustration of being in a profession that is struggling in South Carolina, but I have heard similar comments and observations across the providers in this study—where very few are doing well and even fewer think the Joint is good for chiropractic medicine in general.

THE JOINT'S REJOINDER

In interviews with officials from the Joint as well as with chiropractors who work there, some of the complaints and criticisms made by chiropractors were addressed. In addition, many of the criticisms of the chiropractic profession were discussed, including the training chiropractors receive, the business model they are taught to implement, and how the internal strife of the profession often prevents chiropractors from achieving their goals.

As a starting point, I wanted to learn more about how officials at the Joint see their role and purpose. Here's what one franchise owner had to say about the sublux theory and the Joint's scope of practice:

> The vast majority are Sherman and Life grads around here. . . . And they get real defensive when you ask them, as a non-science person, explain the sublux theory to me and show me how it works . . . and the variability of that across providers. I don't disagree that there's something wrong, because there's pain. What you're calling it, maybe we're getting into semantics, which makes ortho guys crazy because it's not a dislocation. . . . But how do you explain to the public how you are going to fix it? . . . If you're pain management and we can relieve the symptoms, and we're good. But don't say you're going to fix my kid's asthma by adjusting his back three times a week. When people ask me what we do, my first thing is we're not curing cancer or heart disease. We are taking people who have issues with back pain or neck pain and extremity pain and we are putting them on a maintenance program that will either prevent that or reduce the incidence of that dramatically. That's what we do. It's a manual manipulation. And that's all. And it's one of the reasons I could buy into the Joint, philosophically, not just financially. We know what we do and what we don't do. . . . We are not about promoting, don't take vaccines, don't think we cure asthma . . . are there kids who get adjusted and their asthma is better, sure. But we don't promote that. Everything we're about is about living a healthier more active life because that's what we're trying to do. . . . Fifty percent of our treatment is not just about the adjustment, but about the doctor talking to the patient about those things that are causing those subluxations or whatever you want to call it, those issues . . . if that's the way they are sitting on their wallet in the car, or whatever. Those things that cause it aren't going away so we're just giving them an affordable way to keep those things from really causing bigger problems.

Here's what one franchise owner had to say about vertebral subluxations and the Joint's scope of practice:

> When people ask me what we do, my first thing is we're not curing cancer or heart disease. We are taking people who have issues with back pain or neck pain and extremity pain and we are putting them on a maintenance program that will either prevent that or reduce the incidence of that dramatically. That's what

> we do. It's a manual manipulation. And that's all. And it's one of the reasons I could buy into the Joint, philosophically, not just financially. We know what we do and what we don't do. . . . We are not about promoting, don't take vaccines, don't think we cure asthma. . . . are there kids who get adjusted and their asthma is better, sure. But we don't promote that. Everything we're about is about living a healthier more active life because that's what we're trying to do.

The criticism about maintenance plans has an interesting wrinkle. Like many chiropractors, those who believe in the idea of maintenance therapy sometimes frame the discussion in terms of repetitive injuries. This makes intuitive sense, if a patient continues to engage in certain behaviors, such as poor posture as a result of sitting at a desk all day, they increase the likelihood of needing treatment to their back or neck because of that repetitive motion or behavior. Thus, the treatments offered are not maintenance therapy per se, but these are seen as new injuries. If the patient changed their behavior or stopped engaging in that activity, the problems would likely go away on their own and treatment would not be needed. As one franchise owner points out,

> People need regular treatment because of the things you do. People come to us they're injured from working out. . . . Are you going to stop working out? [So is the Joint of the belief that patients need regular treatments to keep the joint and the innate flowing?] No, no, no, no. Nobody ever made guys who believe that stuff follow any scientific rigor. There's a whole lot of people from Haiti that believe if you do voodoo with chickens, that's going to fix a lot of problems, but that doesn't mean it's going to fit with science. What we do serves a population of people. . . . We don't claim to be comprehensive, we claim to be what we are, we're maintenance chiropractic . . . we deal with about . . . if you call and say you're a first timer, one of the question that our wellness consultants ask, "Have you been in an accident in the last two weeks? Have you fallen? What's bringing you to chiropractic care?" If you say you've been in an accident, or "I slipped and fell," we are going to suggest to that they go to a chiropractor first or to their family doctor to get some X-rays done, or we'll send them to the imaging center and they'll ship your X-rays over to us, but we think you need to have that done before you waste your time coming in here. Because we're generally, if we find out in the patient interview, we're generally not going to adjust that . . . and the fifty bucks just isn't worth it.

In response to the concern that chiropractors at the Joint are engaging in unsafe practices or that they cannot possibly diagnose a patient's injuries in the absence of an X-ray, here is what one franchise owner had to say:

> The ACA (American Chiropractic Association) is not convinced that X-rays are necessary, we're following their guidelines. And just putting their hands on people is just not true. Every patient goes through a patient history that are the

red flags for whether they should be treated. And diagnostics . . . for family practice diagnoses are different from cardiac or internist or an OBGYN. The diagnostics are different. So understand that what we're trying to do is determine if that patient is safe to adjust, and to do that the diagnostics are different. . . . And the ACA says most people don't need X-rays and it's overdone, and none of us need more radiation with all the things we have around us.

There are known diagnostic questions and tests that you can determine if someone is safe to adjust or not. They're all taught that in school and they are taught that very well. So they're doing that. The reason you get the criticism about the X-rays, is because this doctor, he graduated and this practice management company told him, you put an X-ray machine in, you can bill more, and Medicare will pay for that. If they quit paying for it, I wonder how long they'd continue to do it. They do the same things we do. So it's a very fake criticism, because it's rooted in money and not in science.

From an operational standpoint, the Joint appears to contain some benefits to working there and there are a number of reasons why a chiropractor might want to become an employee. This one particular franchise owner offers insight into why he tends to hire chiropractors early in their careers. From a business standpoint, it makes sense to hire employees who have some experience in the profession. He says the following:

I generally do not hire fresh graduates . . . for a couple of reasons, number one it takes them a lot of time . . . they do about 250 adjustments while they're there. . . . I can get them that in two weeks. . . . They don't have the skills, there's no internship or residency program, but who wants to lay down on the table and have the intern do the adjustment? But then again, they have the intern doing surgery? But you have to educate your patients and the public about what's going on. Reason number two is that they haven't met reality yet. They haven't lived in the real world. They've been told they're going to make six figures right out of college and they get to us and I'm saying "you're worth about $20 an hour to me to start because I have to pair you up with other doctors to really give you some of the techniques they've learned over the years and that takes me six months to do it. So you're not that valuable to me starting out. Now we can grow that over time depending on how you grow your skills and your dedication and attitude and all those other things." But forty grand is nowhere near the hundred grand they're thinking they're going to make coming out of school. So if I'm going to hire a recent grad, I'm not going to pay him or her what I would pay for someone who has been in the business for a while. Even then, I'm not paying anyone a hundred grand.

This same franchise owner offers insight into the salary structure that he uses to compensate his chiropractors. Consider this observation he makes about the realities of owning and operating a private practice as a chiropractor. He says the following:

> I've interviewed a lot of four-year to ten-year chiropractors. . . . Consistently, 75–80% of them sitting in front of me have had their own practice, and they did make six figures like the colleges told them, which is you make six figures, but you take out all your expenses, this is what you get to take home. . . . And they're working three and a half days a week, because that's what the college told them they should be working. I would say, 80% of them are making 35–45 grand in their own practices, because of the expenses. . . . You go to open your own practice, you got 70 other guys to compete with, the overhead is high, they are opening in the back of other houses in offices that aren't very attractive and they're not mainstream . . . comparatively speaking, I wouldn't have doctors . . . I had one relatively new doctor, a recent Life grad. We had dinner one night, this is about three or four months into it. . . . She's seeing maybe 15–20 patients a day, because she's relatively new and she's the second doctor and patients walk in and want the other guy. . . . They have to build their following, and people who like their style. So we're sitting down at dinner and she pulls out her phone and says, here's what the BLS (Bureau of Labor Statistics) says, $124k a year. And I said, Okay, that's the government, doing what they do best, which is statistics, but in the same way they do everything else, not very well. Because if that were true, how many doctors, I don't have anyone making $125k, how many would be working for me if that were really true? If the average out there, why would they come to me? I can't afford to pay someone $125k, I want to pay them more. I tell them I want, my goal in life is to pay them as much as I possibly can, because if I'm doing that, I'm making money. I've got to have my part too. . . . I've got millions invested in this, I've gotta have my part too.

It is a fair statement that chiropractors, like doctors in general, did not go into their profession with a goal of running a business. I have interviewed many doctors, who have said they want to practice medicine, not run a business. But it is a necessary evil unless they work for a hospital or some other organization that handles that aspect of the profession. It is fair, then, to state it is likely that chiropractors are no more adept at running a business than physicians, and some of the challenges they face in operating a private practice are generated by what they were taught in chiropractic college. As Jerry, a franchise owner of the Joint, and a veteran of owing and running several large businesses, points out, there is simply a lack of any meaningful understanding of what is needed to be successful. He says the following:

> This is why these guys go to practice building seminars, because they don't have the first idea how to run a business. And they take the advice of these guys because it makes sense and they see the dollar signs long before that seminar is over. But even just running a business, it takes some time and effort and you have to monitor what's going on. But these guys are so anti-data that they won't even use tools that optimize their profit. If there was ever an incentive for them to pay attention to that, it has to be the money. So when you talk about

> the two-hour lunch and the half days here and there, there's some truth to the physicality of the profession, but what they haven't done is what you noticed, is why don't you guys get together? They don't build any bonds or relationships with fellow chiropractors and work out the business side of things. . . . These guys don't have any data about how their business is doing, they don't collect any of that important information, and they don't know how to use it to make their business better.

Jerry also points out that his model is really more of a reflection of market demands than what chiropractors are expecting to happen. Like the new chiropractor who was complaining about the low salary, as if Jerry was somehow shortchanging her, Jerry's answer is simple. He says the following:

> The other thing, is that over the course of five years, I have full-time doctors and the fill ins, I have lost two in five years . . . that goes back to compensation, goes back to the way you treat people, and one of them stayed in town here and is practicing in town with another guy, the other guy couldn't sell his house and couldn't handle the commute. So he bought a practice closer to home. . . . So I think it says about the environment I've helped them create, I try to stay out of their way and give them autonomy. . . . But if the compensation was really that bad, why would so many stay for so long? I could be a tougher manager and make more money. . . . There are things that go through the cracks and I let some things go. . . . But what's the long term vs. the short term gain? I would have more turnover, the patients would see it. . . . It's just not worth it to me. But I think if I was paying people too little, they would not want to work for me. Then I would have to respond with a better deal for them. But they keep coming, they stay, and that tells me that I'm right where I need to be. It also tells me that the notion of the private practice is likely on the downward trend. So many of these guys find out they can't make it on their own or they are putting in far more time than they want to—so it's easier to just come work for me—they won't make as much but you know what? They already aren't making as much as they think and they are already working harder than they want to . . . at least I give them the predictability of a paycheck and the autonomy of treating patients the way they think they should.

A representative of the Joint had this to say about the criticisms levied at him by chiropractors and others in the profession:

> We brought 65,000 patients to chiropractic who had never seen a chiropractor before. And what we're doing is making it so accessible and so affordable that people will try it. So for me, it's doing the least invasive, least risky procedure to help you get someone out of that pain. And thankfully, in the last five years, even the American College of Physicians and now the FDA just last week, are recognizing and putting out statements that chiropractic and acupuncture

should be more available. . . . The FDA just said doctors need more training in chiropractic and acupuncture for their patients in the treatment of pain, because this opioid epidemic has just gone crazy. Some of those patients will likely stay with us, but some might consider going to another chiropractor if that provider offers specialized treatments or something we don't offer. I'm okay with that and chiropractors should be thrilled that we are expanding that 14 percent of people who use chiropractic treatments—but they're not.

They're complaining that we are somehow ruining the profession and making it harder for them to function. We are in some ways, we're doing what they don't want to do—stay open longer, we don't take three hour lunches and make it hard for people to find us and we don't claim to cure cancer, asthma, autism, or any of a hundred other problems chiropractors tell patients they can fix. We tell people who we are, what we do, why we do it and make it as easy as possible for people to decide if they want to use us. . . . And we don't mandate maintenance plans. If someone wants to come in and pay each time they come, we're okay with that too. So we're not exploiting patients. So how am I the bad guy in this story? I'm the bad guy because I'm doing what they won't do and they don't like it. Toughen up and decide to do the same thing or don't. But don't blame someone for doing a better job at your profession than you're willing to do.

In discussions with chiropractors, even some who currently work for the Joint, the issue of litigation is a topic of concern. Many believe that some of the parameters of the operational model of the Joint will inevitably lead to injuries by patients and, consequently, lawsuits. In response, one franchise owner had this to say about lawsuits:

You're going to get sued, I don't care who the doctor is . . . you're going to get sued. . . . And we've been sued, it's a matter of public record. And the insurance companies say it's cheaper to settle, so it just creates a vicious cycle because it prompts people to keep doing it. We're pretty tough on the insurance companies, we don't do the go-away money, because that's part of protecting the brand. We follow standard industry guidelines and operate just like any other chiropractor in terms of the decision to treat or not treat, and there really isn't much difference in what we do compared to traditional chiropractors, except we do it more efficiently, more conveniently, and more honestly.

THE JOINT AS DISRUPTIVE INNOVATION

As was mentioned, much of the chiropractic community has a negative perception of the Joint and its presence in the marketplace. While the narrative is largely based on a concern that the Joint is not practicing safe medicine, some observers debate if that is really the main thrust of the argument. Instead, some participants in the study point to the fact that the negative feedback about the Joint stems from the fact that they are meeting a need in the market that current chiropractors are unable or unwilling to address. This is not an uncommon reaction to a new presence in an industry, particularly one that has created for itself a particular paradigm of understanding and operation and one that has not been required to modify its focus.

One way to conceptualize the presence of the Joint into the chiropractic marketplace is found in a theory that was developed by Clayton Christensen (1997). In his book, *The Innovator's Dilemma*, he argues that some innovative creations occur by leveraging technology to enhance a particular product (improving the old way of doing things) or by creating an entirely new market and new sets of customers.

One challenge to understanding the notion of a disruptive innovation is the confusion between this term and a technological enhancement, or what Christensen refers to as a *sustaining innovation.* The latter term refers to improving on existing products. An often-cited example of disruptive innovation is the development of personal computers, which created an entirely new market. Prior to their development, customers who bought computers were usually hospitals and universities because they were so expensive. Thus, innovations occur when a new dimension of an industry is created.

A more recent example occurred when Netflix moved its operation toward streaming of movies on the Internet when much of the industry was still renting physical DVDs in stores in neighborhoods. Such a decision was risky, but it also revolutionized the movie watching industry. Similarly, Google promises to create autonomous self-driving cars, Amazon will likely capture how consumers grocery shop, as they have recently bought Whole Foods. Similarly, 3D printing will likely change the way manufacturing occurs.

The fascinating aspect about disruptive innovations, says Christensen, is that they tend to initially attract customers as unproven and unrefined processes. As a result, these products cannot command a high price. But over time, and with refinements, the companies engaging in disruptive innovations can actually begin to integrate mainstream customers, even the ones relied upon by existing companies.

Also of interest is the initial reaction by companies in industries where there is the beginning of a disruptive innovation—many companies view this new competitor as inferior or question the ethics or quality of the products or services. As a result, the existing companies are slow to respond to these changes because they do not feel the upstart company poses any threat. Slowly, as the new company or product improves, they begin to attract customers and ultimately reshape an entire industry.

Christensen points out that all established companies in an industry must wrestle with making a choice between incremental improvements in existing processes and products or taking the leap and trying to create new markets by adopting new business models through the use of new technologies. This, he says, is the *innovator's dilemma*. For those that focus on doing the same things with minor enhancements, they run the risk of being usurped by an upstart company with a new and better model. For example, long-distance phone calls were fundamentally changed with the introduction of Skype, as was the entire music industry when iTunes allowed users to purchase only those songs they wanted instead of the entire album. They also were able to stream the songs to their iPhones instead of carrying a Walkman or other device in addition to the phone.

In an article published in the *Harvard Business Review*, Christensen offers insight into the problems of disruptive innovation in the health care system in the United States. Many of the tenets of his theory are easily seen in the health care crisis and how incumbents within the system are not interested in changes that greatly enhance the overall health care model in this country. For instance, Christensen points to the fact that the specialization in medicine and what is being taught in medical schools around the country mean there are fewer providers available to treat the kinds of patients with routine and easily diagnosed problems.

So while the medical profession has escalated its ability to deal with unique and rare problems, all at a considerable cost to patients, the routine problems that patients have often go untreated. Moreover, a somewhat odd development has occurred in medicine, where primary care physicians have an incentive to not refer patients to a specialist as they promote continued care in their offices because that is how they are reimbursed (Christensen et al., 2000).

Christensen also points to the fact that laws and regulations have been used in health care to ensure that innovations are contained and controlled to maintain the status quo. A chain reaction occurs when regulators are unwilling to approve certain devices or products, which then trigger the insurance companies, who will not reimburse for the use of a device or piece of equipment. This, in turn, means doctors will not use it because they will not get reimbursed for it, all resulting in patients receiving substandard care and little in the way of improvements (Christensen et al., 2000).

Christensen also points out that some of the changes in health care, such as the use of nurse practitioners and physician assistants, who can easily diagnose and treat routine illnesses and injuries, are currently being prohibited from doing because physicians fear that their value will supersede those of doctors. As Christensen correctly points out, physicians should not be reluctant to provide nurse practitioners and physician assistants with this type of training and authority, as it allows doctors to focus on other aspects of medicine and more critical patients (Christensen, 2000).

Thus, the health care crisis in this country is ripe for a disruptive innovation, but the existing parties that stand to gain from maintaining the status quo are unwilling to recognize its significant value to patients and to providers in the long- or the short run. Part of the reason is territorial—where physicians feel as though their turf has been encroached upon, and part of it is financial, where existing institutions stand to lose significant investments in equipment and for products and services that were, at one time, on the cutting edge of technology. This reluctance to embrace change has a host of negative consequences for patients and for the health care system as a whole (Christensen et al., 2000).

What is happening in the chiropractic industry with the introduction of the Joint can easily fit into Christensen's ideas about a disruptive innovation as well as his thoughts about the resistance to it in the health care industry as a whole. As Christensen points out, initially the incumbent companies discount the value of the new company, by making reference to inferior quality and perhaps safety concerns about the product. As we saw, many in the chiropractic profession question whether or not what providers at the Joint are doing is safe because of the lack of a traditional in-depth diagnosis, complete with X-rays, and an elaborate consultation that usually requires the patient to return the following day for their first treatment.

Christensen also points out that initially, the startup company cannot command a high price for their product or services, in part because it may be an unknown quantity in the market or perhaps refinements are needed to customize the product or service. The Joint bases much of its model on a discounted cost of treatment in an effort to attract a new segment of the chiropractic market. The goal is to offer simple adjustments for $29 for each visit or $59 per month for up to four visits per month (at a per visit cost of about $15), and they are proud of the fact that they have attracted nearly 65,000 new patients who had never previously seen a chiropractor in 2016. Thus, much of what Christensen describes as part of this disruptive process can be seen in the strategies of the Joint.

In response, many chiropractors have complained about the Joint's presence in the marketplace, but have been unwilling to respond in any meaningful way to this new method of operation. Similar to Blockbuster video or the telephone company with the introduction of Netflix or Skype, chiropractors run the risk of remaining steadfast in their adherence to a traditional method of operating, and losing patients in the process due to their unwillingness to adapt to the new opportunities in the marketplace.

While this may make it more difficult for chiropractors to remain in practice, largely because they are already struggling to survive financially, additional time will be needed to remaining open during extended hours, refraining from three-hour lunch breaks, and reducing the price for services, not to mention the apprehension many chiropractors have expressed about going to a cash-only model (which is the one the Joint uses). These changes may end up causing some chiropractors to reconsider whether it is worth continuing in practice. This may be why, as Jerry points out in his experiences with hiring and retaining chiropractors, so many come to work for him and remain employees—either instead of having their own practices or in addition to operating one.

DISCUSSION

Thus, it appears that the Joint is narrowing the scope of treatments they provide and are quite clear on what they will and will not do in terms of treating patients. As one franchise owner points out, while much of chiropractic care centers around treating victims of automobile accidents, that is not the patient pool on which the Joint concentrates its efforts. He says the following:

> We're not going to replace a chiropractor who works with someone who works with auto accidents. . . . That's 80% of their business, and I'm being conservative. . . . Every one of them you interview, you ask them if they were truthful, where do they get their new patients, it's from lawyers. . . . They get a base of lawyers, and they learn how to work that system. Now there are guys that are different in that they take these types of patients, but they don't feed off them like their bread and butter.

There are several issues worth mentioning as we consider the chiropractic profession's response to the Joint. Most people are reluctant to change and the medical profession is no exception—as was mentioned in the last chapter, doctors have a certain understanding of illnesses and prefer to treat patients in a certain way. While as scientists they must remain open to new developments and research that may suggest a better way of treating their patients, there are times when doctors cling to a particular protocol, even in the face of new evidence.

A similar tendency seems to be occurring with chiropractors as they examine what is happening with the Joint. That is, chiropractors have been trained in a certain model of treating patients that involves a certain protocol, involving X-rays, operating a practice with certain features and hours of operation, and many continue to use those methods despite the fact that many chiropractors complain about the loss of patients, increased competition among providers, the use of practice-building seminars that focus on maintenance plans, and the inability to get patients to regularly return for office visits and treatment.

As Jerry pointed out, the ACA, the largest advocacy organization for chiropractors in the world, has taken the position that X-rays are not necessary to properly diagnose a patient. Moreover, the Joint's position is that they are delivering treatments for routine problems that patients encounter. They are not performing traction or electric stimulation, or massage therapy on patients. They are taking a patient history, learning about the problems the patient is having, and following industry protocols to treat them by licensed chiropractors, trained at regionally accredited institutions.

From the accounts provided and the level of negative emotion surrounding the presence of the Joint in the marketplace, it appears that the concerns about safety are not likely the problem. Many of the chiropractors in this study offer the observation that their fee for service is very competitive, particularly in those affluent areas where patients do not seem to mind paying upwards of fifty dollars or more out of pocket for treatment. The introduction of the Joint, however, is forcing chiropractors to rethink how they might operate. As one chiropractor lamented,

> We have tried opening for a short time on Saturdays but no one showed up. So why should I give up my Saturday only to find that no patients are coming in anyway? [How long did you stay open?] We were open from 9am to 12pm on Saturdays. [How long did you engage in the extended hours?] We did it for about a month or so. [Were patients notified or did you have the staff let them know when they came into the office?] Well, we put it on our Facebook page and we had the staff tell those patients who came in, but it just never caught on, so we stopped doing it.

This was not a good strategy for this provider, for many reasons, and it demonstrates a fundamental lack of understanding of how businesses need to operate in order to be successful. One cannot simply post a message on social media and let only those regular patients know of the extended hours. In all likelihood those regular patients prefer the schedule they are on—the goal is to either invite new patients or those patients who might not be able to visit the office during normal business hours. But these likely never knew about the extended hours because the practice did not really notify them.

The fact that many providers are only available three days a week to begin with, along with three hour lunches, despite the complaints about a failing practice, is a curious development. The introduction of the Joint, however, readily calls attention to this issue. They are open well past normal business hours, they are open on weekends, one does not need an appointment, and their prices are lower than every other chiropractor in town. It is no wonder that the chiropractic community is concerned about their presence. As one chiropractor pointed out, "they are eating my lunch!" He's correct.

But instead of responding as any other business in a competitive market would, by extending their hours, launching their own innovative marketing plan, or offering some type of unique treatment or service that the Joint is not providing, the chiropractors in this study appear to be content to reframe the discussion into one about patient safety. While this may deflect questions about what chiropractors are actually doing to improve their practices, one wonders why there is much of a concern in the first place.

In a profession that embraces independence and autonomy, and in a marketplace that rewards innovative thinking, the person who provides the better service at a cheaper price is going to be more successful most of the time. If people in that market are not happy about their current state of affairs, they have the opportunity to change it. Some will, but many will likely continue to complain or simply accept their fate as factors something beyond their control. If chiropractors are that concerned about patient safety, why are they not collectively organizing and attempting to respond to the threat companies like the Joint represent? Why are they so angry about the Joint but are unwilling to address other providers who represent a much greater threat to their credibility and legitimacy in medicine? Remember, the Joint hires licensed chiropractors and does not allow them to perform a wide range of treatments. Thus, it appears that chiropractic medicine is experiencing a disruptive innovation and time will tell what chiropractic care looks like in the future.

But this volume-based approach is essential for the Joint's business model to work. It is a bit ironic that some of those same chiropractors who are critical of the Joint use the same justification in their own practices for the use of maintenance therapy, but real questions remain about whether such treatments are needed to maintain a healthy lifestyle or the patient's overall health. Beyond regular exercise, proper nutrition, periodic checkups (at six-month or one-year intervals for most things), and with the exception of brushing one's teeth twice a day, there are few things that require weekly treatments to keep a person healthy. If the individual feels better and wants them, such as getting a massage every week or so, and can afford it, that's one thing. But even the regular massage is not going to improve a patient's health—it might make them feel better or relieve symptoms, but its actual impact is limited.

NOTE

1. Interestingly, some of the same complaints levied by chiropractors about the Joint are nearly identical to what the medical profession has claimed about chiropractors.

REFERENCES

Christensen, C. M., Bohmer, R. M., and Kenaghy, J. 2000. "Will Disruption Innovations Cure Health Care?" *Harvard Business Review*, September/October. Available at https://hbr.org/2000/09/will-disruptive-innovations-cure-health-care

English, C. and Keating, E. 2015. "Majority in U.S. Say Chiropractic Works for Neck, Back Pain." *Gallup*. Available at http://www.gallup.com/poll/184910/majority-say-chiropractic-works-neck-back-pain.aspx

"Health consciousness among baby boomers could boost demand for chiropractic." 2011. *Chiropractic Economics*, November 1st. Available at https//www.chiroeco.com/health-consciousness-among-baby-boomers-could-boots-demand-for-chiropractic

Lisi, A. J. and Brandt, C. A. 2016. "Trends in the Use and Characteristics of Chiropractic Services in the Department of Veterans Affairs." *Journal of Manipulative Physiological Therapies* 39: 381–386.

Long, P. H. 2013. *Chiropractic Abuse: An Insider's Lament*. New York: American Council on Science and Health.

Magner, G. and Barrett, S. 1995. *Chiropractic: The Victim's Perspective*. New York: Prometheus Books.

McMillen, M. 2011. "Complementary and Alternative Medicine on the Rise." *WebMD,* available at https://www.webmd.com/a-to-z-gudies/news/20110201/complementary-and-alternative-medicine-on-the-rise

Russell, J. 2015. "Walk-in Chiropractic Clinics Aim to Expand a Slowing Industry." *Chicago Tribune*, November 19th. Available at http://www.chicagotribune.com/business/ct-chiropractors-clinics-11-20151119-story.htm

U.S. Department of Labor, Bureau of Labor Statistics. 2016. *Occupational Outlook Handbook 2016-2017 Edition*, Chiropractors. Available at http://www.bls.gov/ooh/healthcare/chiropractors.html

Why the Joint is an Attractive Business Model. The Joint.com. Available at http://www.thejointfranchise.com/research/joint-attractive-business-model

Chapter 6

Chiropractic Colleges

One of the most critical dimensions of chiropractic medicine involves the training providers receive in performing treatment on patients. As we have seen in previous discussions on scope of practice, the varying philosophies of chiropractors influence what they think they should be doing when patients visit their offices. Recall the common typology to classify chiropractors: Straights, Mixers, and Reformers. This typology is driven, primarily, by the training chiropractors receive and their subsequent objectives in the treatment of patients.

In addition to understanding the various philosophies of chiropractic medicine, there are a host of issues that stem from students' experiences while attending chiropractic college. Included in this discussion is the high cost of obtaining a degree, student debt, which plagues most college students, but particularly chiropractic students, the lack of training in operating a practice, as well as the absence of residency programs for chiropractic students and loan forgiveness for those who dedicate their time to underserved populations.

Many chiropractors in this study, particularly graduates who attended their program within the past ten years, complain that they were not prepared to meet the demands of starting and running their own practice and feel as though they were misled when informed of the starting salaries they could expect upon graduation and licensure. To be fair, one could argue that these issues present challenges for all students, but the problem seems more acute for chiropractic students given the significant debt they carry upon graduation.

Chiropractic colleges, which are typically stand-alone institutions and not affiliated with a larger university, also face the challenges found in a changing higher education landscape and wrestle with declines in enrollment, rising costs, administrative accountability, and efforts to discover an acceptable level of sustainability in the future. There are also accreditation issues, the controversy over which relates to the internal strife within the profession and its future.

While it is impossible to know for certain whether the chiropractic community is fragmented because of differing ideas about the profession or because of the many philosophies that are found in chiropractic colleges, the end result is that the profession remains beset with internal challenges from which it may never recover.

As one dean noted earlier, if a person went to a dentist in Europe and then again to one in the United States, they would likely receive very similar types of treatments for a toothache. Similarly, if a person sustained an injury and needed a physician, while there are a host of different ways to solve that particular problem, there are some standards that all physicians would start with and progress along some logical path toward recovery. Not so with chiropractic medicine, which is noted for its wide range of ideas on how to diagnose and treat illnesses and injuries. It seems fair, however, that some of the responsibility for this divergence must be borne by the schools that train students in chiropractic medicine.

With only a few exceptions, chiropractic colleges fall under the Carnegie Classification of Institutions of Higher Education, Graduate Instructional Programs, private not-for-profit, with a special focus of four-year health professions schools. This essentially means they are designated as schools designed to train students in a particular area (health professions) and are considered doctoral-level institutions (Carnegie Foundation, 2014). This designation differs from research-oriented doctoral programs that train students who wish to enter the academic profession.

The Carnegie classification provides a framework for educational and research purposes where it compares institutions that are similar in format and purpose. The framework only includes all accredited, degree-granting colleges and universities in the United States that are reflected in the National Center for Education Statistics Integrated Postsecondary Education Data System, more commonly known as IPEDS (Carnegie Foundation, 2014).

The Carnegie Classification system was created by the Carnegie Commission on Higher Education in 1970 to standardize information about colleges across the country and allow meaningful comparisons of data for research purposes. In 2014, the responsibility for collecting this data was assigned to the Center for Postsecondary Research of the Indiana University School of Education. However, the Carnegie name has remained the same (Carnegie Foundation, 2014).

While fourteen of the sixteen chiropractic colleges are classified as doctoral programs for a specific field, two exceptions to this classification are D'Youville University, which only recently launched a chiropractic program, and the University of Bridgeport, which has a doctoral program in STEM fields. Both of these institutions have embedded their chiropractic medicine program into an existing university and have created a separate college or school on campus. This is an important consideration because for many years, chiropractic colleges in the United States were unsuccessful in formally collaborating with a university.

According to their website, the University of Bridgeport's College of Chiropractic have not been submitting data to IPEDS about its students. Repeated requests for an interview with the provost and the dean of the College of Chiropractic Medicine were unsuccessful, so the only information available about its program comes from its website. D'Youville's dean was very helpful in explaining the program and its goals. Similarly, Keiser University launched a new College of Chiropractic in 2017. Like his colleague at D'Youville, the dean of that program was a resource in understanding the larger issues in chiropractic education as well as in articulating the goals for its program. However, because two of these programs are new, limited information about them was available.

Some colleges who submit data on its chiropractic program include aggregated data from its institution, meaning information about its chiropractic program is included with data from all of its graduate and undergraduate programs of study. This results in a limited ability to conduct an individual assessment of its chiropractic program.

This chapter begins with the discussion of the training that chiropractors receive by examining the philosophical differences of the chiropractic colleges, along with issues relating to enrollment and accreditation issues within the profession. Other topics include the cost of attending, residency programs, student loan forgiveness, and the preparation students receive for life after graduation.

DIFFERENT PHILOSOPHIES OF THE COLLEGES

As was mentioned, there exists a wide range of philosophies among the chiropractic colleges across the country. A few, such as Sherman College of Chiropractic, are very clear about their philosophy. This is highlighted by the clarity of their mission statement, its core values on the institution's website, as well as in interviews and conversations with their provost, campus historian, and the Director of Evidence-Informed Curriculum and Practice. Sherman's mission statement reads: The mission of Sherman College of Chiropractic is to educate and prepare students to become doctors of chiropractic.

This mission is based upon the college's core values and is achieved through activities in the areas of education, research, and service. The core values of the institution more concretely define its philosophy. They are as follows:

1. Integrity and ethical conduct are critical to all aspects of college operations and to maintaining professional relationships with constituents including students, patients, employees, the profession, and the public.
2. The health needs of patients are supreme and central to the doctor of chiropractic program and critical to establishing trust between doctor and patient.
3. The clinical practice of chiropractic focuses on the location, analysis, and correction of vertebral subluxation.
4. The college honors its long-held traditions that teach respect for the innate intelligence of the body and the inseparable and synergistic nature of the philosophy, science, and art of chiropractic.
5. The college community actively seeks and promotes advanced learning and exploration of ideas relative to the college mission in an environment of respect and academic freedom (https://www.sherman.edu/mission-statement/).

Similarly, Life University has a specific statement of purpose. According to its website, the mission of the college is this: "Our purpose is to provide students with the vision to fulfill their innate potential, the inspiration to engage in a quest for self-discovery and the ability to apply a principled approach to their future roles as leaders in humanitarian service and as citizens in their communities."

Vision Statement

Our goal is to maximize the expression of the perfection within.

We recognize

that all organic systems in the universe are conscious, self-developing, self-maintaining, and self-healing.

We believe

that these systems work best when they are free of interference.

We understand

that the nervous system is primarily responsible for orchestrating the internal and external dialogue of the body necessary for life.

We acknowledge

that there are three interferences to the nervous system: physical trauma, environmental toxins, and emotional stress.

Therefore, our purpose is to correct these interferences, allowing the organism to express its innate potential.

Of critical importance is our Doctor of Chiropractic degree, which is focused on the relationship between the spine and the nervous system and the aberration, called vertebral subluxation, as well as its detection and correction, allowing a greater expression of the perfection within (https://www.life.edu/about-pages/president/mission/).

Life West University Parallels Life University's vision statement, which says the following:

> Life Chiropractic College West offers a doctor of chiropractic program through a leading edge curriculum and clinical training experience providing graduate chiropractors with the knowledge, skills, philosophies, attitudes, and competencies is to serve the health care needs of the public in the 21st century. The program focuses on the relationship between the structure and function of the human body as coordinated by the nervous system and the effect of the vertebral subluxation. The program instills in the chiropractic graduate an appreciation for the innate potential of the human body to heal and adapt to its environment and the role of the nervous system in the restoration, preservation and enhancement of human health and performance. The Doctor of Chiropractic program prepares graduates for personal and professional fulfillment in a climate of loving, serving, and giving. (http://lifewest.edu/about/mission-statement/)

Of all the chiropractic colleges in the United States, these are the most detailed mission statements. All three identify themselves as institutions that strongly believe in vertebral subluxations and the Innate. Clearly Life, Life West, and Sherman would be classified as "straight" schools and their philosophies are integrated into the training of its students. Other colleges offer more general statements about its mission. Consider the Texas Chiropractic College mission statement:

> Our mission is to promote excellence in the education of practice-ready doctors of chiropractic who are focused on evidence-informed, patient-centered care; seek new knowledge through scholarship and research; and engage our communities through ongoing service. (http://www.txchiro.edu/student-services/about-tcc/mission-statement.html)

Such a statement contains all the current key phrases used in the field to show that the institution is interested in a scientific approach to chiropractic medicine. The phrase *evidence-informed* or *evidence-based* suggests that the college takes into account empirically validated principles and treatments rather than adhering to tenets of the past, which lacked scientific proof that chiropractic treatments were effective. Some of the information contained on the Texas Chiropractic College website suggests a belief in vertebral subluxations and its treatment, but unlike Sherman or Life, there are no references to the Innate concept.

At the other end of the spectrum, The Los Angeles College of Chiropractic, as part of the larger Southern California University of Health Sciences, has a reputation, at least among the chiropractors interviewed for this study, for endorsing a Reformist philosophy, even though this can only partially be determined from its mission statement. It says the following:

> Our mission is to education students as competent, caring, and successful integrative healthcare practitioners. The University is committed to providing excellence in academics, service, scholarship and leadership through the Los Angeles College of Chiropractic, the College of Eastern Medicine, and the College of Science and Integrative Health. (http://www.scuhs.edu/academics/los-angeles-college-of-chiropractic/)

This mission statement contains another key phrase used by chiropractors in the profession, particularly those who see chiropractors as primary care providers. The word *integrative* is used quite frequently in the literature to describe chiropractors who wish to work as part of a health care team of providers to offer comprehensive treatment to patients. However, this mission statement could be used to describe almost any program at the university and the initial sentence could describe virtually any college with a health program. Similarly, Northwestern Health Sciences University's mission statement is even more broad. While anecdotal evidence from interviews with officials from the university indicate that they subscribe to a Reformist approach, nothing in their mission statement indicates this as their philosophy in chiropractic medicine. Their mission statement is as follows:

> Northwestern Health Sciences University prepares the next generation of healthcare professionals to delivery and advance health care. (https://www.nwhealth.edu/get-to-know/mission-foundation-statement/)

Such a statement does not, by itself, identify the college's philosophy or what they attempt to teach its students. In fact, only a few of the chiropractic colleges are clear about who they are and what they are about; most contain general statements that do not offer much in the way of insight into the college or university's identity much less how they perceive their role in chiropractic medicine.

In fact, a review of all the chiropractic college's websites, particularly their mission, vision, and philosophy statements, found that most mission statements mention the idea of a sound education, and usually included phrases like integrity, commitment, dedication, and the like, but most are so generic that they could be used to describe almost any educational institution.

This was a curious development during the study and in the interviews with academic leaders at many of the chiropractic colleges, I asked about their specific institution's philosophy and the possible reasons why it is so difficult to discern their stated philosophy. While most of the deans and provosts demurred about their own website, claiming they did not have control over its content and often gave very general descriptions of their respective college's philosophy, some deans offered the idea that a stated philosophy or public identity was too controversial for many chiropractic colleges.

Steve, a dean at one of the chiropractic colleges, who is attempting to change the school's identity to one that focuses on a more integrative approach, said that this transition is not an easy one and progress remains slow and controversial. He talks about the impact that the alumni have on the public position of his institution, who do not want to be labeled with a particular paradigm or philosophy. He says the following:

> There are so many schools out there, Bob, that are just afraid to put anything specific in their website. They are so afraid of offending their alumni, you know the guys who are very vocal but don't really donate any money. But they complain about anything they think might affect the image of the school. These guys are crazy, but the schools respond to it. So I think one of the reasons you can't find any meaningful statements about a given school's philosophy, aside from the Life's and the Sherman's, is because they purposely keep things very generic. They don't want to offend anyone by having a mission statement that could be interpreted as putting the school in a box. Are they Mixers, are they Reformers, or are they something else? This is another example of the infighting we've talked about in the profession. But when you start involving the schools in the discussion, then the problem gets even bigger.

Other reasons for this lack of an obvious proclamation about the philosophy of the school may be related to recruitment. As Amy, a dean at a chiropractic college, points out,

> I'm not sure a lot of chiropractic colleges want that information made public. It could hurt recruitment efforts. If prospective students want a more integrative approach and there is Parker or Texas, or some other school saying they are not, then that student will immediately move on to another school. In this day and age of declining enrollments, every student counts so perhaps some of the colleges don't want to make that information so easily known. Maybe their admissions people want an opportunity to talk to students so they can have a chance to convince them that their school is the better option. Sort of like when you visit a car dealership while shopping for a new car, they don't want you simply calling and asking for a price. They want to get more information about you and have a chance to make a pitch.

While it may be a bit disturbing to campus officials to think that they are mentioned in the same breath as car salesman, perhaps this dean has a point. It is not clear whether or not the omission is intentional for recruitment purposes, but after reviewing all the chiropractic college websites, it seems very difficult to identify the main differences between chiropractic colleges just by obtaining information online or in brochures, admissions materials, or even by talking to admissions counselors.

Jack, another dean, offered the observation that many chiropractic colleges, like universities around the country, are struggling with their institutional identities. In the changing landscape of higher education in general, and with the heavy criticism of chiropractic medicine in particular, some colleges may be moving in the direction of a more integrative approach, but are not quite ready to define themselves that way. He says the following:

> What you may have encountered are schools that don't know who they are or what they want to be. The profession is in a state of flux and can't figure out who they are, so why would we think the colleges that train them are any different? In fact, I'd say that the colleges and their lack of understanding of the need for unity ARE the reason we are so divided as a profession. The Palmers and the Shermans and Life are all wrapped up in their dogma and the rest of them are trying to emulate physicians, which is just as bad in my view. No one is ever going to consider chiropractors primary care physicians and we aren't going to be seen as specialists like Osteopathic doctors. But the buzz word of the day is "evidence-based practice" so all are moving in the direction of trying to prove that what it is we do actually works. It does, it's just that we don't have the data to prove it. So a lot of the colleges are using the terminology of science and medicine and trying to act and sound like doctors. Of course, we can't make the Shermans and the Lifes and the Palmers go away, as much as we might like to do that, but it also means there are lots of different schools teaching very different techniques.

As an illustration of Jack's point, Ed, a dean at a Chiropractic College, offers this standard account of what he tells people about how his college trains its students. He says the following:

> There are three main things that we try to stress to students. Everything chiropractors do with a patient is pretty much the same as an MD, until they get to the treatment. We do our history the same, we do our physical exams the same, we're using standard models, of how to evaluate a patient. Where does it differ? If you're coming in for low back pain, I'm not going to send you through a drug pathway, unless you need it. There are times when you need it. I'm not going to send you for surgery, unless you need it. There are times when it's needed.
>
> But 90% of the time, back pain has a muscular skeletal component and a psychological component. We talk about it a lot. And most of our treatment in

> chiropractic, we have spinal manipulation, we have soft tissue therapies that we do and we have cognitive behavioral aspects we have to address. And some of that includes lifestyle counseling, stress counseling, if you have a lot of stress, it actually activates the pain pathways. We train our students a lot and say, "Hey, if you have a patient, especially a fibromyalgia patient? A lot of that is coming from that third intervention." I'm not saying do cognitive behavioral therapy as a chiropractor, we're not trained for that. But be able to recognize that there's a lot of mental stress involved in this, we need to get this patient some thought therapy, in addition to the muscular skeletal issues. Because they all contribute to back pain, and dysfunction.
>
> So that's the approach we're trying to push. We're just scratching the surface on what spinal manipulation is doing as well. But a lot of their work involves, let's say you hurt your knee, how does that change the pathway into the spine. . . . We actually can note changes at the dorsal root level, which is at the base of the spine, but also there's feedback coming down from the brain that actually causes changes to those pathways as well. So that's why sometimes a muscular skeletal injury can actually lead to depression. You'll see that in surgical cases as well. Patients that have open heart surgery have really high incidences of depression . . . because the pathways change. . . . It has the most sensory input in the body. We try to tell students, "Don't forget that words are also sensory input . . . and that can actually change their muscular skeletal system." We're just scratching the surface to understand these connections, it's not as simple as moving a bone back in place, which, by the way, we don't do . . . the freeing up the Innate.

A related problem occurs when a college attempts to modify its philosophy but has not made the evolution to a more integrative approach. As Ed points out, there are operational challenges to consider as well as philosophical ones. He says the following:

> There are integrative models that we are trying to build. . . . Now are we perfect? No, there are still faculty who buy into the dogmatic models and reject the ideas of evidence informed ideas, so you can't just blow it up and start over again. . . . You need to do this over time. When I was brought in, it was to invite a change to the curriculum, the one used in Scotland. . . . And they are learning foundational science while learning clinical science. A lot of med schools are using this spiral curriculum and we are probably one of the only ones . . . how to get faculty involved. . . . So we're looking at specific competency . . . in a competency-based system, we can know exactly what students learned when they are done with the course, and prove that they've done that . . . and faculty can't really validate that . . . assessment drives learning. . . . So it should be an interesting couple of years ahead for us. The deans in the schools are talking about the evidence-based, competency-based models, we need students who are critically thinking, not just what some charismatic teacher told them and taught them some techniques.

Another dean talks about the criticism that integrative chiropractic colleges confront with regard to diagnosing patient problems. Critics point out that chiropractors are not sufficiently trained to treat a wide range of illnesses and believe that the adjustment is the answer to every problem. Dave, a dean at one of the integrative chiropractic colleges, says the following:

> We tell our students "Don't be afraid to refer and don't be afraid to treat" . . . and that's basically our philosophy. . . . But we still need to know how to diagnose, because if a patient comes in with diabetes, and how many overweight patients don't know that they have diabetes, so if we sent them to have blood sugar levels, to determine if they have diabetes, they're going to respond better than someone who comes in and just gets adjusted. Hypertension, etc. although we don't treat them, they are responding to our treatments once we know what's going on. . . . And we have to be smart enough to develop treatments or refer out when it is out of our scope, based on that knowledge and the only way we can do that is to be able to diagnose.
>
> I hope we're getting the message out that we are an evidenced-based program that graduates doctors of chiropractic that can work in any environment, whether it is private practice, group practice, hospitals, military, so on and so forth. Our graduates can earn the trust of others in the health care fields, and we want them to be able to speak the language of modern science, we want them to be critical thinkers and not be led astray by bizarre philosophies or cult-like ideas that have been a part of the old chiropractic profession. So we're wanting to make a clean split with them. And we've even gone so far as to get away from the idea of bone displacement in the spine.

As a justification for the use of a more integrative model in training chiropractors, one college official pointed to research where chiropractors were used as first-line responders to patient needs. Jim, a dean at one of the chiropractic colleges that espouse a more integrative approach, says the following:

> I think it was the AMI study about five years ago, in Illinois I think, Chicago, where they actually used chiros as primary care first line physicians . . . where they were triage doctors. . . . And the patients would come to the chiros first, and they would evaluate them. And if they could treat them they would, and if they needed referral they would send them to the docs that were involved in the study. And apparently, it saved the state like $400 million a year. You should really look at that study; it was a profound study.

Many of the colleges that espouse a more integrative philosophy are also distancing themselves from the notion of the vertebral subluxation. Part of this has to do with gaining credibility within the medical profession and part of the reason stems from a commitment to proving the effectiveness of spinal manipulation. As Tony, a dean of an integrative chiropractic college, states

> You know, the big fight in the profession is that our accrediting standards are taking subluxation out of the standards, the term "subluxation." . . . I mean most of us call it an "intersegmental dysfunction," because we know there's something wrong with the joint. But it's hard to prove an actual subluxation. If there's pain in that joint, there has to be dysfunction in that joint, or there wouldn't be pain. So pain over that capsule itself would make it an intersegmental dysfunction. . . . Those are easily provable.
>
> The sublux theory becomes a pivot point for those discussions of the identity, because the sublux is the bread and butter of chiropractic . . . so to do away with that we are doing away with our identity and so is the lack of internal consistency . . . so many colleges with different ideas.

ACCREDITATION BATTLES

Tony's comments raise an interesting point about chiropractic colleges and their philosophies. The issue of accreditation, an essential piece in chiropractic education, has itself had a long and stormy history between the colleges and its accrediting body, the Council on Chiropractic Education. The issue of whether or not chiropractors should serve as primary care physicians or whether there can be more than one dimension to chiropractic medicine has been debated for years. The debate escalated significantly when the CCE decided to delete particular terms from the standards used to assess chiropractic colleges.

Specifically, the terms *vertebral subluxation* and *drugless* were removed from the definition of chiropractic medicine in the CCE's standards of policies and procedures. Such a decision was, ostensibly, designed to broaden the profession's parameters to include chiropractors as primary care physicians and to advocate for prescription drug rights for chiropractors. Such an act, however, resulted in a firestorm of controversy, since, as Tony points out, the term *vertebral subluxation* is the "bread and butter" of chiropractic medicine. In order to understand the significance of this decision, along with the conflict between some chiropractors and CCE, some context and history is needed.

Essentially, the Reformist approach, which spearheaded the idea of training chiropractors to be more like physicians, complete with prescription drug rights, was seen as a response to a declining overall market for chiropractors, spurred by decreasing reimbursements from insurance companies and declining enrollments in chiropractic colleges. Thus, the notion of chiropractors being trained to think and act more like physicians came as a result of the profession's inability to sustain itself only as providers who treat neck and back injuries with chiropractic adjustments. Such a position, however, was felt by many conservative and traditional chiropractic groups, such as the Straights, to be a betrayal of the core tenets of the profession and would result in a fatal blow to chiropractic medicine's distinctiveness.

In response, these traditional and more conservative chiropractors accused Reformists of contributing to the overall decline of the profession. This controversy naturally included how chiropractic students were being trained, since some chiropractic colleges were in support of this approach and their curricula reflected this integrative model.

As McCoy (2012) points out, the problem really began around 2002 when a number of articles in the *Journal of Chiropractic Medicine* focused on the issue of prescription drug rights for chiropractors as well as the conceptualization of chiropractors as primary care physicians. While initially much of the controversy went unnoticed, a group of chiropractors began to see these efforts as part of a much larger and coordinated effort to redefine the profession.

Some observers of this trend even went so far as to consider this a conspiracy within the profession, referring to those who supported the changes as the "Chiropractic Cartel." This cartel consisted of several chiropractic organizations, including The CCE, the National Board of Chiropractic Examiners (NBCE), the Federation of Chiropractic Licensing Boards (FCLB), the ACA, The Congress of Chiropractic State Associations, and several chiropractic colleges (McCoy, 2012). While prescription drugs were the specific topic, many observers argued that this was the proverbial tip of the iceberg. What the Cartel really wanted, they said, was to redefine chiropractors as primary care providers with the goals of enhancing the reputation of the profession, improving revenue streams, and addressing enrollment challenges at chiropractic colleges around the country (McCoy, 2012).

The CCE was established in 1971 when the ACA separated itself from its Council on Accreditation. There were, at the time, two accrediting agencies, the CCE and the Association of Chiropractic Colleges, which were supported by the International Chiropractic Association. Since neither could claim to represent the entire profession, neither qualified for recognition by the United States Office of Education, now the U.S. Department of Education. As Kent (2012) points out, the two groups could not agree on many important issues and many state chiropractic associations would only accept licenses from CCE-accredited schools.

While both groups wanted the federal government to identify them as the accrediting body for chiropractic education, the CCE went forward with their application first and it was approved by the U.S. Office of Education. The FCLB passed a resolution that its state board members revise its bylaws for licensure that applicants show evidence that they had graduated from a chiropractic college recognized by the CCE. These events effectively provided CCE with the authority it needed to decide on matters relating to chiropractic education (McCoy, 2012).

Many conservative chiropractic groups believed that CCE would attempt to eliminate Straight chiropractic by restricting efforts by chiropractic colleges who espoused this philosophy. This led to a series of lawsuits, primarily by Sherman College of Chiropractic and Life University. In 1979, Sherman College brought a claim in federal court against the U. S. Commissioner of Education's renewal of CCE status as a federally recognized accrediting agency for chiropractic colleges. The Court found that not only was the CCE adequately represented the profession, but the ideology of Sherman College was "the doctrine of a deviant splinter group" (McCoy, 2012, p. 15).

In that same year, Sherman brought a complaint to the U.S. Department of Justice against the CCE, arguing that the CCE conspired to restrain competition within the chiropractic profession and education. This investigation found no evidence of any illegal action. Two years later, in 1981, Sherman College and the Straight Chiropractic Academic Standards Association (SCASA) filed an antitrust suit in District Court against the ACA, claiming the CCE conspired to restrain Sherman and the SCASA's ability to compete in chiropractic education. They also claimed that the CCE abused its authority as the only accrediting agency by colluding with state licensing boards and the FCLBs to exclude Sherman graduates from the profession. The Court rejected Sherman's claim and ordered Sherman to pay the court costs (McCoy, 2012).

In 1988, the SCASA petitioned the U. S. Department of Education for accrediting status as an alternative to the CCE. This was approved, but CCE challenged SCASA's authority in California, claiming the SCASA did not act responsibly in maintaining high academic standards for its chiropractic colleges. Coupled with Sherman's loss of accreditation by the Southern Association of Colleges and Schools, the U.S. Department of Education revoked SCASA's accrediting authority in 1993. Sherman then applied to the CCE for accreditation, which was granted in 1995 (McCoy, 2012).

Similarly, Life Chiropractic College received accreditation from CCE in 1985 but encountered sanctions from the CCE from the outset, particularly philosophical disagreements with CCE over diagnosis and case management. In 2002, CCE revoked Life's accreditation as a chiropractic college. In 2003, Life filed a lawsuit against the CCE claiming among other things, that CCE had adopted standards for its chiropractic program that unfairly discriminated against the Straight chiropractic philosophical approach. Life's suit was successful and the two sides reached an agreement that allowed Life to state that it has continuously held its accreditation since 1985.

In 2012, critics again attacked CCE for its decision to omit key terms in the definition of chiropractic medicine: *vertebral subluxation* and *drugless* as it applies to the definition of chiropractic medicine. These modifications were said to further erode the traditional understanding of the role of chiropractors and the ability of Straight chiropractors to operate within the profession.

In 2011, the U.S. Department of Education's National Committee on Educational Quality and Integrity (NACIQI) held a hearing to consider renewal of CCE's authority. Both sides in the debate, traditional chiropractors, supported by the International Federation of Chiropractors, the Foundation for Vertebral Subluxation, the Movement for Chiropractic Quality and Integrity, and the International Chiropractic Association, lobbied against the CCE and its leadership. Similarly, the ACA and the Association of Chiropractic Colleges supported the efforts of the CCE, claiming in part that there have been improvements both in the quality of chiropractic education as well as in the performance of students on licensing exams who have graduated from CCE-approved colleges.

As a result of a considerable lobbying effort by traditional chiropractors, the NACIQI reported forty-two violations of recognition criteria in their report, most of which were administrative in nature. Committee members directed the CCE to show compliance with one particular section of the Recognition Criteria: 602.13, which deals with the wide acceptance of the standards, policies, and procedures within the profession, and to demonstrate how its standards advance the quality in chiropractic education. This particular issue is crucial to the complaint filed by the traditionalist.

This group claimed that the change in standards and policies was designed to change the mission of chiropractic medicine from a specific and limited domain (one that contributes to patient health by the correction of vertebral subluxations) to that of a primary care physician. This is significant since many states define chiropractic as a form of medicine that is limited in scope to specific areas of the human body, namely the spine and neck. Further, the classification of chiropractors as primary care physicians is incongruent with many state laws that identify chiropractors as those who are trained in the removal of vertebral subluxations. To remove the term, they argue, is to negate the conventional and legal understanding of what chiropractors are allowed and trained to do.

In response, in 2016, the U.S. Department of Education gave CCE one year to address all of the violations of the recognition criteria and to demonstrate that there is widespread support for its standards, and, perhaps most importantly, that its policies actually improve chiropractic education. Given that a vast majority of the forty-two violations were administrative in nature, this was thought to be a rather routine matter. The latter violation, however, is unlikely to be resolved, given the strong division within the profession and its inability to agree on fundamental issues. As of this writing in July 2018, the CCE report has not been released. Tony, a dean at one of the chiropractic colleges, points out that this debate has a significant impact on how chiropractic colleges will function in the future and the incompatibility between the two groups about the direction of the profession.

> And then when CCE, our accreditors, took out subluxation and drugless profession out, the Straights filed a complaint with the U.S. Department of Education. . . . They pushed to the point where our accrediting body nearly lost its right to accredit. It gets pretty intense, instead of someone saying "Let's paint a broad brush and you put yourself where you think you want to be inside that picture," they just want to draw the dot and "this is where everyone needs to be." And there's no room for real compromise if they are wedded to one dimensional definition.

As Tony points out, such intractable positions reverberate throughout all aspects of the profession. Likely the reason for the deletion of the term *drugless* relates to the desire of many Reformists to advocate for prescription drug rights, even though most advocates of this approach want a limited scope of authority—to include only muscle relaxants and anti-inflammatory drugs. Given that many chiropractic offices already contain over-the-counter versions of these medications (such as BioFreeze cream), including many Straight chiropractors' offices, Reformists may have a point.

The reason for the elimination of the term *vertebral subluxation* is likely due to the fact that the scientific community has not seen evidence that subluxations actually exist and that chiropractic treatments are proven methods of correcting them. This gets into the debate about what constitutes proof and data, as was discussed in the chapter on scope of practice. Given that there does not exist definitive proof, many Reformists are, as one dean pointed out, distancing themselves from such an ideological position since it threatens the credibility and survival of the profession.

In sum, there is an obvious connection between the varying philosophies of the chiropractic colleges around the country and the dispersion of ideas about the scope of practice among chiropractors. It seems reasonable that one's training generally informs the types of treatment a given provider considers appropriate for patients. It is also clear that the division between Straights, Mixers, and Reformers is reflected in the profiles of the chiropractic colleges. The fact that there is no common ground and that the infighting calls attention to the fact that there remain questions about validity of the profession could explain why so many colleges are seeing declining enrollments, why the colleges demure on articulating a stated identity, and why so many chiropractors are experiencing difficulty in sustaining their practices.

ENROLLMENT ISSUES AND SUSTAINABILITY

Perhaps the most reliable and accurate source for information regarding the enrollment trends for chiropractic colleges in the United States is the IPEDS data. IPEDS is a series of surveys conducted by the U.S. Department of

Education's National Center for Education Statistics. IPEDS collects data on every college that participates in the federal student financial aid program, a mandate of the Higher Education Act of 1965. Information must be reported about a wide ranges of trends, including enrollments, graduation rates, finances, student financial aid, and about faculty and staff, among other variables. More than 7,500 institutions complete IPEDS surveys each year (National Center for Education Statistics, 2017).

According to a 2013 study of data from IIPEDS chiropractic college enrollments have remained stagnant or in decline for a number of years. More recent analysis of IPEDS enrollment data shows that this trend has continued through 2015, the most recent data available.

As Figure 6.1 shows, the 2013 study showed that enrollments at chiropractic colleges were at its highest levels in 1996 when enrollments peaked at 15,390, and witnessed a significant drop between 1996 and 2002 when it bottomed out at 9,709. Since then the enrollment figures have remained flat or fluctuated only slightly, about 1 percent or less, for each year until 2013 at 9,863. It was during this time that two chiropractic programs closed, the Colorado College of Chiropractic and Cleveland College of Chiropractic-Los Angeles.

D'Youville University launched a program in the early 2000s and Keiser University launched a new program in early 2017. Despite these new programs and attempts by other chiropractic colleges to open satellite campuses in other cities around the country, more recent IPEDS data reveals that enrollments decreased about 1 percent between 2013 and 2015, at 9,767,

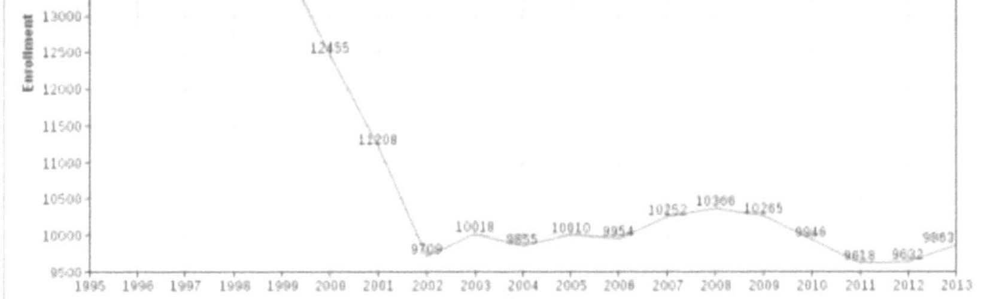

Figure 6.1 Declining Enrollments At Chiropractic Colleges 1995–2013.

demonstrating a continuing problem for chiropractic colleges all across the country (see Figure 6.1).

While the data seems gloomy for chiropractic colleges, like all colleges and universities, some will be better able to weather this decline over time. However, the reality is that what chiropractic colleges are experiencing with their enrollment is similar to what many graduate programs are encountering.

According to the Council of Graduate Schools, a Washington, DC-based advocacy group for all graduate programs around the country, enrollments have remained stagnant at many graduate colleges around the country, with the aggregated data showing only modest increases in enrollment since 2014. Generally speaking, most experts argue that graduate enrollments are often tied to the strength of the economy, where enrollments increase when the economy declines. For example, during the recession in the United States in 2009, when many employees lost their jobs and had to rethink their careers, enrollments in graduate programs increased dramatically. Obviously, being laid off is a motivating factor in retooling in one's career and given the absence of jobs in the marketplace, many people decided to return to college to earn a graduate degree in the hopes of being more marketable in their chosen or related career. Others likely decided to start over and begin a new career. As the economy recovered and unemployment declined, so did enrollments in graduate programs across the country.

As of 2015, enrollments have shown only modest improvements as the economy has remained strong and there is less concern about career changes or enhancements. Moreover, there are several impediments that prevent a large proportion of graduate students, particularly at the doctoral level, from completing their programs of study. The Council points out that the costs of attending are considerable, as are family constraints, and the time it takes to compete a doctoral program.

The Council estimates that the attrition rate for doctoral students is as high as 50 percent in some programs of the study. The loss of academic jobs, particularly those that carry with it tenure as a benefit, is also disappearing. Thus, the attraction of an academic career does not hold the same level of opportunities as it had in the past, which can also influence the willingness of doctoral students to make the commitment, time, and expense to complete a program of study. As officials at the Council of Graduate Schools point out,

> Between the fall of 2010 and 2011, first-time graduate enrollment fell 1.7%. This was the second consecutive decrease in such enrollment since the fall of 2003. This decline was not only in fields one would expect such as education, but also in engineering and other STEM fields. In the past international students could be counted on to fill the gap, but preliminary estimates from a CGS survey of international student applications for the fall of 2013 indicate that

> the numbers from key countries are trending down. For example, applications from China, which in the past has accounted for 29% of international graduate students at U.S. institutions, appear to be down 5% for fall 2013 following double-digit increases for the past several years.
>
> Given the global competition for graduate students it is essential that we find ways to not only reverse the declines in U.S. graduate enrollment but significantly accelerate the flow of domestic students into our graduate programs. And in doing this we know from earlier research that financing is a strong factor in graduate student success. In a recent study of doctoral program completion, 80% of the respondents in an exit survey indicated that financial support was a key factor in their ability to complete the degree. (Council of Graduate Schools, 2017)

While the Council of Graduate Schools indicates that enrollments are increasing at modest levels and contain high attrition rates, chiropractic colleges appear to be quite different; with declining enrollments and higher completion rates than many other doctoral-level programs. While the Council's estimate is that doctoral students carry an average debt of approximately $50,000 beyond what was owed as an undergraduate, chiropractic college students assume a much higher level of debt, upwards of $200,000 or more.

Another difference between graduate programs in general, even doctoral programs, and chiropractic college enrollments is that the decline witnessed in the data on chiropractic colleges has lingered long before and remained stagnant long after the economic recovery has occurred. As was mentioned, the precipitous decrease shown in Figure 6.1 indicates that the problems began in the mid-1990s and have remained flat since then, with negligible increases for the past decade or more. This indicates a more chronic problem plaguing the profession and it does not appear that the strategies employed by the chiropractic colleges have been successful.

Perhaps the declines in enrollment are a result of alumni, as the marketplace ambassadors of the programs, who have experienced significant adversity in terms of their own success, have not attempted to recruit students as they have in the past. As many chiropractors in this study have pointed out, they are quite reluctant to encourage anyone to enter into the profession, particularly since the return on the investment, given its significant costs, has been slow in developing. As Doug pointed out in one conversation,

> I don't think I can ethically tell someone to consider going to chiropractic college. I mean, I had a good experience at Sherman, but the industry has changed, the profession is completely screwed up and the money simply isn't there in adjusting people any longer. And the number of people, at least in this area, is crazy. I like my colleagues and all, but at the end of the day we are all in competition with each other. That hardly breeds a sense of community or comradery.

> So given the cost, the lack of success, and the amount of time you have to dedicate to this, why would I consider telling someone to do what I did? I know a lot of guys who say they won't be encouraging their kids to go into chiropractic, and that used to be how many of them ended up there—they had a parent or an uncle who was a chiropractor and they seemed to be successful. I see now that this might have been in another era, when people got reimbursed for what they did, but I also see how tainted this profession has become as guys have gotten so desperate and are willing to compromise so much of their integrity to stay afloat.

Some deans and provosts offer insight into a changing demographic to explain the enrollment challenges in their respective institutions. As Jack, a dean at a chiropractic college, points out,

> I think the nature of students has changed. I know the students we attract are not the philosophic ones. In my interviews with them, I want good evidence-based critically minded students who can lead this profession somewhere. Life University might as well be an entirely different profession because it seems like they are only interested in collecting more religious converts than anything else.

Joe, a successful chiropractor, points out that he thinks the types of people who apply to chiropractic college are those who cannot get into medical school. Joe says the following:

> You got guys now who don't have a shot at getting into medical school and now they think they can get in through the back door by going to chiropractic school. The problem is, even those schools who say they are training primary care providers, they aren't training doctors. They may give them more courses on diagnostics, but in the end, they aren't in medical school and everyone knows that. And the kids coming in today think they are going to be treated like doctors, but they're not and nobody really thinks of them that way, no matter what the college is telling them. I'm a supporter of my chiropractic college even though it was thirty years ago. Do I think we want to be seen as an institution that takes all the rejects from medical school or those people who couldn't get in even if they wanted to? No! That hurts the profession and it hurts the college. But if we don't stop this nonsense about calling chiropractors primary care physicians we are all going to be out on our asses because no one will believe that we can do anything well.

Joe's comments about the enrollment challenges facing many chiropractic colleges seem to be related to the scope of practice issues discussed in earlier chapters. Joe is suggesting that the shift to a more integrative approach by many chiropractic schools will not only negatively impact the entire profession, evidence of the wisdom of such an approach is seen in lower enrollments.

In conversations with recent graduates, however, they seem to offer a slightly different view, regardless of the philosophy of the chiropractic college they attended. Whether a Straight school or Reformist, many of the younger chiropractors were attracted to the lifestyle benefits of chiropractic medicine. As Kathleen points out,

> I never wanted to go to medical school. I think I could have gotten in because my grades were good, but when I thought about all that doctors do, especially those that aren't specialists, between the hassles of running a practice, the lack of reimbursement, the amount of time I was going to be spending on call or going to the hospital, I thought, "why would I want that?" Instead, what I found, or thought I found, was that chiropractors didn't have to do all of that and could maintain a lifestyle that was conducive to doing the things I wanted to do. I mean, a three day a week schedule and making six figures? Who wouldn't want that? I also wanted to help people and thought I had the personality and talent to get them better, which is why I became a chiropractor and an acupuncturist. But medical school? That just wasn't what I wanted. And given the way medicine is playing out, talk to those guys about how satisfied they are—most of them think of themselves as pill pushers not doctors. I didn't want any part of that. So I'm not sure that answers your question, but I think the chiropractic schools are trying to be like doctors and it isn't working—their enrollments aren't improving at all. I'm not sure if that's because the kind of people who want to be chiropractors don't want to be doctors so they're not going to chiropractic college or if it's something else.

The realities for chiropractic colleges are that enrollments have remained flat and only a few colleges are witnessing increases in enrollments. Like other colleges around the country, officials at chiropractic colleges are looking for ways to expand enrollments and to maintain a consistent student population. While other colleges and universities are attempting to build revenue streams through online initiatives or to build partnerships with community colleges and other collaborations, chiropractic colleges remain stand-alone entities. Even those colleges who have a clearly defined philosophy and purpose are struggling to meet enrollment goals. In only a few cases, such as Sherman College of Chiropractic, one of the smallest chiropractic colleges in the country, enrollment growth has occurred. As the provost, Dr. Robert Irwin, noted,

> From my perspective, each institution is approaching it (enrollment challenges) from their own perspective. Trying to identify how they can attract more students. A few years back the Association of Chiropractic Colleges had a discussion on the trend and came up with some strategies to boost overall interest and enrollment in all chiropractic colleges but I don't think it got much traction and, as you can see the trend has not changed with the exception of a few schools improving and fortunately Sherman is one of them.

Unlike other colleges, many chiropractic colleges are not embracing the idea of online education. Dr. Irwin states his views about Sherman's involvement with online education:

> Sherman is not at this point. There are a few courses what would lend themselves to being online but we don't have the data that indicates that the students would prefer it or that it would have any impact on enrollment. And as you point out, our courses are very hands on and also the ones that are not, such as biochemistry, still have a great deal of integration with other courses that having them taught on campus just makes sense at this stage.

Internal data from Sherman, the only chiropractic college in South Carolina, indicates that they have indeed run counter to the general trend of declining enrollments. As outlined in Table 6.1, enrollments at Sherman have improved in the last five years. The number of students in 2016 was 384, which is slightly lower than that in 2015 but larger than the student population during the years between 2005 and 2014, when many other chiropractic colleges sustained significant decreases. The recession likely had a significant impact on this trend, as the entire country was severely impacted, particularly during 2007–2009. However, Sherman appears to have sustained considerable growth since 2012, where enrollments have returned to their 2002 levels, at just under 400 students.

While there may be some variation in marketing strategies among the chiropractic colleges, most employ standard admission counseling approaches, with open houses, social media, and traditional campaigns to attract students. Further, the strategies used when prospective students contact a chiropractic

Table 6.1 Sherman College of Chiropractic Enrollment Trends

Year	*Enrollment*	*Percent Change (%)*
2002	376	—
2003	480	21.6
2004	434	−9.5
2005	372	−14.2
2006	330	−11.2
2007	289	−12.4
2008	240	−16.9
2009	201	−16.2
2010	184	−8.4
2011	189	2.6
2012	237	25.3
2013	286	20.6
2014	346	20.9
2015	391	13.0
2016	384	−1.7

college appear to be the same—follow-up calls and emails and attempts to personalize the experience for the student are now standard practices for all colleges and universities that use a computerized platform that tracks calls, contacts, and delivery of materials to prospects. In an attempt to explain Sherman's resurgence, the provost of the college notes that its clarity of mission is likely the driving force behind Sherman's enrollment success. He says the following:

> Well, Sherman is enjoying a steadily growing enrollment in the last four years and the projections are looking very favorable as well. We attribute it to doing one thing really well from a program standpoint and that is focusing on improving health through the traditional approach to chiropractic as opposed to diversifying into other programs. We seem to have found our niche while other schools are struggling for an identity. In addition, it is not, nor has it ever been, our desire to be the biggest, but we want to be the best and so we are putting our energy into program improvements. We are starting a campus renovation project to ensure up to date facilities that reflect the quality of our program and to accommodate our projected growth.

In some ways, perhaps there is an important point in these observations: the continued internal strife within the profession and its inability to define itself could be resulting in students being hesitant as they do not necessarily know what they are getting from a particular chiropractic college, particularly if it is not clear about its mission or purpose, and the information from its websites does not clearly define them. While there are a few chiropractic colleges that have not wavered in their institutional identities, Sherman stands out as a fixture in the chiropractic community.

While others may disagree with this stance or consider it dogmatic, Sherman has not wavered in their beliefs about chiropractic medicine and that may be attractive to students. Life University, another chiropractic college that has a clear sense of purpose and institutional identity, has not had the same level of success in enrolling chiropractic students however, so ideology is clearly not the only factor prospective students consider in making a decision to attend a particular chiropractic college.

MICROLEVEL ANALYSIS OF THE CHIROPRACTIC COLLEGE EXPERIENCE

As was mentioned in the previous chapter, most chiropractors, like physicians, did not enter their chosen profession with the idea of running a business. As one doctor put it,

> I didn't go to medical school to run a practice. I went to medical school to practice medicine. I'm not good at running a business and I don't really want to—what I want to do is what I do best, which is to treat patients. But I can't do that the way I want to if I don't have my own practice. So I do my best to get good guidance from people who know how to run a business, but medicine is a little different than selling traditional services or products.

This was a consistent message, whether it was an interview with a physician or a chiropractor. Some are naturally gifted and take to operating and managing a practice, while others struggle with the financial and mechanical aspects of running a business, such as hiring staff, marketing, compliance with state and federal laws, and so on. Because it is a central theme in medicine, this was a topic of discussion during the interviews with chiropractic college officials as well as in accounts from practitioners about how they fare with this dimension of the profession. One main conclusion drawn from these discussions is that there exists a disconnect between what the chiropractic colleges think they are providing students and what graduates say they need in order to be successful. For instance, here is what one chiropractic college official had to say about what their particular institution offers. Jim says the following:

> We bring in outside practitioners in whenever we can. . . . We actually have a lot of Canadian students so once a year we bring in an entire panel of Canadian chiropractors and from the licensing board, and insurance, and they spend like three hours with them. We have also initiated the billing and documentation class. Once they graduate from school, they no longer document the way that they should. . . . So we have a course on billing and documentation that while they are treating patients, they do it appropriately so that the treatment aligns with the codes and what services they provided. All of our clinics have EMRs [electronic medical records] now, so they know what to expect when they get out . . . the clinics look like any other practice. . . . And we actually have a national compliance person who looks at that since we use those problems as teaching moments when it doesn't work.

Many of the colleges offer a course in starting and running a practice. This course often requires students to submit a business plan, similar to what would occur if they were applying for a loan from a bank. Other colleges include visits to existing practices in their local community that are owned and operated by alumni, so that current students can see the many different ways chiropractic offices function. Despite the fact that these courses exist, some chiropractors say they are still ill-prepared when the time comes to begin the process. As Kat, who does not have her own practice after working in the profession for three years, says,

> I had that one course that everyone talks about in chiropractic college. But I don't feel it gave me all that I need to be ready to open my own practice. Not that I think I want to at this point because I can't afford to do it with my loans. But it was kind of a blow-off class—you went through the motions but they didn't really ask a whole lot of you. Given that there are a million other things on your mind at that point in your program, you usually take the course near the end, you are paying attention to so many other things that none of it really stays with you.

While this may be an issue that centers on the amount of effort dedicated to the course rather than the course content, Kat's comments were consistent with other chiropractors who were part of the study. As Melissa points out,

> Hey, I wanted to know more about how to run a practice. I have a background in English, so I don't know the first thing about running a business. But the school only offered one course. And it didn't really help to prepare me for what was coming. I had no idea what I was doing. I bought all this equipment, went into serious debt in addition to my loans. Now I don't think I'll ever get out from under it. I know now that it was a rookie mistake—I should have bought used equipment and only what I absolutely needed, but they also told me that image counts and that I should look professional and polished. Well, how do I do that with crappy looking equipment and in a place that looks run down? This is what I mean—they don't tell you the things you really need to know about how to get started and stay successful. This is why all those practice building seminar guys make money off of us. . . . We don't know how to do it and the school just dropped the ball with it—and I kept hearing "don't worry, you're going to make a lot of money so it will be a challenge in the beginning but you'll get it all back." That's such a load of crap and it's deceptive and underhanded. Why not just tell me what I need to do and be honest about it? Don't most small businesses fail? Why set me up for failure like that?

Other chiropractors mention both this lack of awareness of how to operate a business and a realistic sense of what the market really looks like. Graduates, particularly recent ones within the last five years, complain about what they thought their careers would look like upon graduation and the stark reality of it shortly thereafter. Many talk about having to work multiple jobs, including shifts at the Joint, bartending, and other employment, just to make ends meet, let alone open and sustain a practice.

The comments offered by providers in this study are consistent with the research that has been conducted on this dimension of the chiropractic profession. In a 2011 study that surveyed alumni from eleven different chiropractic colleges, when asked to rate their preparedness for operating a practice, respondents gave an overall rating of 2.02 on a 5-point scale, with 5 demonstrating "Well Prepared." Moreover, researchers in this study examined this trend over several years and found that this finding had not changed since the earliest data was collected in 2004. That year, the average score was 1.94 (Foundation for Vertebral Subluxation, 2012).

On the college side, some deans have pointed out that this is consistent complaint from alumni, but wonder what they can realistically do about it. As Amy points out,

> Let me go back to when I was at Northwestern. I think we had about 3.5 credits on instruction on billing, etc. and the alumni surveys were across the board, we love the faculty, etc. but the business education sucked. So we set out to develop a whole new curriculum called business and ethical foundations. And we had focus groups and ended up with 13.5 credits, in the first semester . . . differences in personality, business practices, which is basically 11 or more credits more than anyone else had. So fast forward a few years, the alumni surveys said the same, thing, love the school, love the faculty, but the business education sucked.
>
> So when I came here I thought I knew what the missing link is . . . video lectures, what they need to do is get out into doctors' offices. We have a number of credits later in the program for understanding things like billing, etc., marketing, what they need to get started. What we do differently here, we get our students out in doctors' offices right from the second or third week from when they start in school in that first semester. We have a network of doctors locally. We send them to a different doctor each semester, but we want to eventually engineer it that they can do a different doctor every eight weeks. Some doctors have them sit at the front desk, some want them to help with history, all sorts of things. But the experiences are coming back are incredible.
>
> Some of my students have been to two or three different offices and have a collection of models of what they want or don't want to do. I don't think anyone else is doing that. While they are getting their academic learning, there are a list of objectives that they are fulfilling with these other offices. I have them do a reflective essay at the end of each semester that demonstrates to us what personal growth they have experienced. . . . One guy said a doctor gave the student homework . . . and he had them go to the mall and observing customer service perspectives by some of these companies in the mall. They get it way earlier in their careers.

While Amy offers some constructive changes that integrate a kind of externship learning that allows students to observe how practices operate, there remains the issue of how much is enough. Amy designed the course sequence so that it began early in the student's time in the program and consistently exposed them to a variety of issues. As she points out, the feedback has been more positive than in the past. It seems that what students are saying they need is more than a single course or even a year-long course in how to run a practice. What they need is firsthand exposure and mentoring from existing chiropractors on some of the challenges they will face.

Unfortunately, when this was mentioned in the interviews with college officials, many deans and provosts thought it was a good idea but did not think they would integrate it into their curriculum, citing time and resource constraints. Others stated that part of "paying their dues" as a chiropractor was learning how to do things for themselves and that it was not the responsibility of the college to teach them how to be successful. Such an extraordinary remark raises questions about what officials think they should be doing, particularly given the costs of attending chiropractic college. As Jim, a dean at one of the chiropractic colleges, points out,

> It's my job to get them ready to understand how to treat patients. It's also my job to give them the tools they need to be successful. But these Millennials feel such a strong sense of entitlement that they don't want to work hard to succeed. Maybe it's good that we don't spoon feed them everything. A little bit of adversity is a good thing. . . . It builds character and teaches them to learn from their mistakes. So it is reasonable in my mind to give them a course on how to run a practice, but I'm not there to serve as a free consultant if they do things incorrectly either. I have only so much time to teach them how to treat the patient, which is the most important thing. No one showed me how to run a practice when I got started. That's what working for a chiropractor is for. They learn the ropes, pay their dues, and yeah, maybe they get exploited by that chiro for a while, but it teaches them things you won't find in a book.

Costs of Attending and Debt

Many of the chiropractors who participated in this study, particularly those who have graduated in the past ten years, talk extensively about the cost of their education, particularly in light of the salary they are making. Given that these providers are still paying on their student loans, coupled with the inability to generate significant revenue from their practice, this is a salient issue for them. The issue of costs and debt incurred by chiropractors also likely contributes to the sense of desperation some feel when they consider diversifying their practice to include other ventures, such as nutritional supplements or weight loss programs. These may or may not be in alignment with a given provider's philosophy of treatment, but the realities of making ends meet only with chiropractic treatments result in some difficult decisions. As Doug, said, "Hey, the need to pay my bills trumps whatever ideology I might have about how I operate a practice."

The costs of one's education and the enormous debt many chiropractors carry, coupled with so many other providers in the marketplace, result in many struggling to succeed. One alternative, of course, is that the chiropractor can moonlight by working for more successful chiropractors, work for the Joint, and engage in other investment ventures, such as day trading or real estate. However, perhaps the most concerning response is to engage in questionable treatments and/or billing to insurance providers.

As Table 6.2 shows, the costs of attending chiropractic college are considerable. Most of the programs are about three years in duration, with some additional time needed to complete all the requirements for the program of study. While most colleges provide an estimate of the costs of attending their institution, not all of them include all the necessary information needed for a prospective student to know exactly what it will cost to attend. This type of information is important in making an informed decision about a particular chiropractic college, but none of the websites for organizations dedicated to chiropractic education offer it. Each student is left to their own devices to determine the actual costs and many do not realize the enormity of the expense until they are too far along into their program of study. As Kat points out,

> Another thing about chiropractic, you spend as much on school as an M.D. does, but you make half the money. I don't think financially, unless you have a giant pile of cash behind you, it doesn't make much sense to become a chiropractor. I looking at what my financial future looks like, it's under control, but was that the right thing to do money-wise? I really like what I do but could I have found something else that cost less and eighth of the price that I would have enjoyed as much. I mean when I got out, I was in about $180,000 and I didn't have any other grad debt. It's a mortgage payment. Especially if I am thinking about opening my own practice.
>
> Folks like me . . . I know a lot of people that . . . now, but people I know that I graduated with like ten years ago, they have an income-based repayment, sort of like a sliding scale, and after a certain amount of time, if you have been making payments consistently, like 25 years, the debt is forgiven, you just have to pay the taxes on it. It's a huge chunk of money or would have paid, unless you make a million dollars a year in your practice and then it's not really an issue. I've had a really interesting time sort of navigating post-school employment.

Kathleen is much more candid in her views of the chiropractic college experience. She thinks the schools take advantage of students by selling them a story and a dream so they will accept the enormous costs to achieve it. She says the following:

> I think a lot of these colleges are pretty predatory, they're all for profit. . . . Knowing what I know now? Would I have gone into it? I mean I like doing what I do and I like helping patients, but at the end of the day I wonder if it was really worth it. . . . This isn't the Mercedes 80s, if it was fifty grand in debt or even a hundred grand in debt, but not what it is now. . . . Is it really unrealistic to start at like seventy grand a year when you have two hundred grand in debt? I don't think it is. I mean I think if you put that much time and money into it you

Table 6.2 Key Data Points by Chiropractic College

College	*Enrollment**	*Graduation Rate (%)***	*Cost ($)***	*Default Rate (%)*	*NBCE (%)*
Bridgeport	N/A	95	195,480	9.2	83
Cleveland	483	80.2	166,866	5.2	91
Life Univ.	2,754	N/A	165,565	10.1	88
Life West	499	90.8	176,085	4.0	89.1
Logan	899	82.8	191,300	2.3	85
LA College	876	78.3	224,742	4.6	81
National	705	82	122,784	1.8	94
NYCC	965	88.6	119,910	0.5****	84.5
NW Health	879	89	169,668	3.0	91.6
Palmer (IA)	1,032	80.2	192,270	2.3	83.3
Parker	977	81.2	205,125	6.7	89.6
Sherman	346	87.5	164,360	2.1	89.7
Texas	260	N/A	154,592	6.5	82
W. States	839	87.5	162,689	2.0	84.6
Keiser	N/A	N/A	N/A	N/A	N/A
D'Youville	N/A	N/A	N/A	N/A	N/A

*2015 figures on enrollment. Other data such as NCBE scores, graduation rate, and length of program were obtained from each institution's website. Default rate on student loans was taken from institution's websites or the U.S. Department of Education database on default rates by institution.

**Graduation rate is determined by the number of students entering the institution as full-time, first-time, degree/certificate-seeking undergraduate students in a particular year (cohort), by race/ethnicity and gender; the number completing their program within 150 percent of normal time to completion; the number that transfer to other institutions if transfer is part of the institution's mission. National Center for Education Statistics.

**When cost of attending figures were not offered from website, IPEDS, or the institution, an estimated $10,000 per year in living expenses was used to determine overall costs. This was used because that amount was what was estimated for living expenses by other chiropractic colleges.

IPEDS data was incomplete because some institutions are not required to submit information. Additionally, some institutions do not offer key data points from their website. Attempts to contact these institutions to obtain said information were unsuccessful. Also noteworthy is the fact that some institutions only offer tuition figures but contain many additional fees.

***New York Chiropractic College only reported default rates on Stafford loans. They did not contribute data to the U.S. Department of Education database.

shouldn't be okay with making twenty grand a year. Doctors make about forty grand a year as residents for goodness sakes.

This sense of feeling misled or even manipulated is a common lament among chiropractors with less than twenty years of experience. It may also explain why so few alumni contribute to their alma mater. Granted, most graduate schools generally struggle with fund raising because there is not the same emotional connection felt in alumni's undergraduate experience, but if many chiropractors feel as though their college has exploited them, why would they give back to the institution? As Janice, a chiropractor who has about ten years of experience in the profession, says the following:

> The information we're given is very deceptive. When you first get into school, you've got people telling you that you can make like a hundred and seventy grand a year. But that's like ten years into the profession, if even then. But you are sucked in and don't know any better. But you don't know what to expect and you're trusting the people there to give you the right information, but they don't. I think it is very misleading. Because you get out and you've got all this debt and a set of expectations of what my career is going to look like and it's not that way at all. . . . So it's a rude awakening when you get out and find yourself having to scramble to make ends meet. They never tell you that while you're in chiropractic school and if they did, I think a lot of people would think twice about going or staying once they got started.

Perhaps Janice has a point—given the enrollment challenges at chiropractic colleges, where most do not have endowments and are tuition-driven, a loss of even a small number of students can have a devastating effect on the college's ability to meet its financial obligation. As was mentioned in previous chapters, the Bureau of Labor Statistics data indicates that chiropractors are generally considered mid-level providers, who are on par with physical therapists, physician assistants, and nurse practitioners with regard to salary. Given these figures, there may be some reason for chiropractic college officials to embellish what the market looks like for students while they are in the program. As Kathleen correctly points out, why would anyone spend close to $200,000 to obtain a job that pays, optimistically, $80,000 per year? Based on the accounts of the chiropractors in South Carolina, few make even that much while being engaged in full-time practice.

In contrast, the costs of attending a medical school are about the same as those of a chiropractic school. In fact, according to the Association of American Medical Colleges' *2014 Medical Student Education: Debt, Costs, and Loan Repayment Fact Card*, the average medical student in the United States graduated with a median debt of $180,000 in 2014, the latest figures available (Becker's ASC Review, 2017). However, the starting salaries for family practice or primary care physicians, according to the Department of Labor Statistics, for 2016 is $200,852 (Bureau of Labor Statistics, 2016).

Aside from the costs, which are considerable, it appears that chiropractic colleges do a good job of getting most of their students through the program in a timely manner. The U.S. Department of Education determines the graduation rate by the number of students entering the institution as full-time, first-time, degree/certificate-seeking undergraduate students in a particular year (cohort), by race/ethnicity and gender; the number completing their program within 150 percent of normal time to completion; the number that transfer to other institutions if transfer is part of the institution's mission (National Center for Education Statistics, 2017). While it is difficult to determine graduation rates for graduate schools in general, and while some programs have attrition rates that hover around 50 percent, many people who begin a chiropractic program of study complete it. Thus, in general it appears that chiropractic colleges do an adequate job of getting their students to complete their programs of study in a timely fashion.

Also noteworthy is the low default rate. Many older chiropractors talk about the "fact" that chiropractors have the highest default rate on student loans of any group. In actuality, according to the Department of Education data, the national average for defaulting on student loans is 11.1 percent. As Table 6.1 shows, none of the chiropractic colleges have default rates higher than the national average and, with the exception of Life and the University of Bridgeport, at 10 and 9 percent respectively, most are below 7 percent. Because other data have been found to be aggregated in IPEDS, meaning both Life and Bridgeport merge their undergraduate and graduate data, it may be that their student loan default data is also included, which could explain the higher rates.

It is also fair to note that students are generally successful in completing their competency exams after completing their program of study. The National Board of Chiropractic Examiners exam is the benchmark for determining if chiropractic students have sufficient understanding of the basic sciences as well as proficiency in the clinical dimension of their programs of study. There are four portions of this exam. In Part I, the exam covers six areas of basic sciences: general anatomy, spinal anatomy, physiology, chemistry, pathology, and microbiology. Each test has ninety standard multiple-choice questions, eighty of which are scored. Each Part I subject is allotted seventy minutes of testing time (National Board of Chiropractic Examiners, 2017).

Part II covers six clinical science areas: general diagnosis, neuromusculoskeletal diagnosis, diagnostic imaging, principles of chiropractic, chiropractic practice, and associated clinical sciences. The same testing protocol is used in Part II as in Part I, with a certain number of questions in a timed environment (National Board of Chiropractic Examiners, 2017).

Part III tests the following nine clinical areas:

- Case History
- Physical Examination
- Neuromusculoskeletal Examination
- Diagnostic Imaging
- Clinical Laboratory and Special Studies
- Diagnosis or Clinical Impression
- Chiropractic Techniques
- Supportive Interventions
- Case Management

In this section of the exam, there are a total of 110 standard multiple-choice questions and 10 case vignettes. Each section is allotted two hours of testing time, with a twenty-minute break between sections (National Board of Chiropractic Examiners, 2017).

Finally, Part IV consists of three major practical sections: diagnostic imaging, chiropractic technique, and case management. Students are asked to visit various stations and review the scenarios, follow the instructions, and perform the required techniques. The Chiropractic Technique section and the Case Management sections are given together and require approximately two hours and forty-five minutes of testing time, but may require an additional five hours of time (National Board of Chiropractic Examiners, 2017).

In terms of scoring, each phase of the exam is scored between 125 and 800 with 500 used as a mean and 100 as a standard deviation. The expectation is that students taking the exam will meet a minimum score of 375 for each part (National Board of Chiropractic Examiners, 2017).

Thus, the NBCE exam is a robust, in-depth assessment of both academic and clinical knowledge of basic sciences and chiropractic techniques. As Table 6.2 shows, the weighted average, or the combined score for the entire exam, for the majority of the chiropractic colleges, is around 80 percent. This means that 80 percent of the students who take the exam from these institutions pass all four portions.

Managing Expectations of New Graduates

As was mentioned, one of the most common laments by recent graduates is the inability to earn a salary commensurate with their level of debt along with the type of job graduates can expect. As we saw with Joe, who is near the end of his chiropractic career, he thinks that graduates come out of college with unreasonable expectations about salary and quality of life. He says the following:

> While some new chiropractors see the practice and where I am, what they don't see is the fact that when I got out of college thirty years ago, I lived in a one-bedroom apartment, I still drove a five-year-old car and I didn't go out to dinner much. I learned the business by working during lunch, I didn't get much in the way of bonuses, because the guy I worked for took advantage of my efforts. Graduates today want to come out of college and think they are going to make six figures. They're not. They want to buy a new car, they want to have nice things, and that's okay. But it isn't the reality they are living in. . . . This Millennial generation doesn't want to pay their dues like everyone does in their profession. They are tired of being poor and think they should have everything handed to them. I tell my new associates, you'll get there but if you want it, it doesn't come easy or quick. They don't want to hear that.

Jack, a dean at a chiropractic college, says the following:

> I think all graduates need to have their expectations adjusted a bit. I'm sure every college advisor or faculty member has to explain the realities of their discipline or profession to potential graduates about what their careers are likely to look like. I would guess that most graduates, who tend to be more ideological in the beginning and more cynical at the end, are found in every profession. Chiropractic students are no different from any other college graduate in that way. I think we tend to get overly optimistic and enthusiastic about what our students are going to do.
>
> But if we are honest, we know about how they will struggle, we know the traps they are likely to fall into, and we aren't really doing a good job of educating them or at least making them aware. And if we are, and then the students don't listen, we can't be held responsible for that. But I don't think we have done enough to get them ready. I will likely be criticized for this from my colleagues, but many of us were also practicing chiropractors before we got into higher education, so we know what their futures look like. Maybe we are just afraid of saying it because it will discourage them and perhaps lead to lower enrollment in the future, but that shouldn't be the reason we don't reveal important information to our students.

Doug points out that the high costs of attending chiropractic college can have a significant impact on how graduates practice, with a risk of some engaging in unethical or questionable practices because they become desperate to earn money. He says the following:

> The other one that I don't know if you're going to get into or have any reason to is the cost of education is a massive one. Because I think . . . I was telling you about some of the shadier things I have encountered, and I think that comes from a sense of desperation, with so much debt over your head, you start panicking and then you start doing stupid things. I do foresee that being an issue as well. . . . It's not like it's going to go down . . . the practical realities . . . finding

a job, starting a practice, or sustaining one. . . . The last time I talked to you, you said you were going to see that other chiropractor . . . and that's one that stuck with me a lot . . . I remember talking to him and I asked him "how much debt did you leave school with?" And he was like fifteen or twenty grand. Now it's like a hundred and sixty grand, and the reimbursements are down so that discrepancy is going to lead to a lot of problems and I don't know what the statistic is, you could look it up, but chiropractors generally default on student loans a lot more than other professional . . . higher education loans. Because I think people come out delusional about what they are going to do. . . . They think they're just going to put a sign on the door and it's just going to happen. . . . I was, certainly, for a bit when I first got out, and then reality kicked me in the face. . . . I think there's a lot of people who have left the profession, guys I went to school with, are now teaching or doing something else, because it just wasn't working for them.

Kathleen goes a step further and argues that many chiropractic colleges misrepresent themselves to students, both in the early stages when a student is selecting a college and near the end when the student is ready to graduate. For her, the entire process is skewed with the goal of taking students' money and not giving them accurate information about their career paths.

When I chose to go back to school for this I looked at the Department of Labor . . . the information is way off . . . even my school, and I wrote them a letter. . . . The average chiropractor makes $99,000. . . . Because in my first year I made like $24,000 and that was a lot more than most people I knew were making. I would love to hear the responses from the colleges. . . . What are they telling grads? I think at some point there's going to be a very large class action lawsuit against the chiropractic colleges. I mean, I would participate in it. There's a lot of misrepresentation. . . . The money, what you'll be doing . . . all of it.

Doug offers this insight into the realities of graduation and starting a career:

And I'll tell you another thing, like for me anyway, I'm not married, I don't have kids, so if it gets skinny, it gets a little skinny. Where I think people went wrong is every class before I got out, maybe a couple of years before, it was unlimited reimbursement. . . . It was a boom. These folks got out, didn't owe much money, were making buckets of money, and they started developing these lifestyles that required it and when that stopped, they ran into binds. I know a lot of guys that had big ass boats, and nice houses and stuff like that and boy it's getting harder and harder every year . . . and like the first two years we were here, still kind of on the tail end of that. . . . It was just starting to come to an end.

Actually the second year we were open we grossed more money than any other year we were open, which is kind of crazy. You would think it would get better, but instead it has kind of hovered and stayed the same, maybe some dips and minor peaks and valleys, but for the most part, that's what led other people to get into other means of supporting themselves or diversifying the practice in

> a way that they wouldn't normally go, like let me bring in an acupuncturist. But for brand new grads, I don't know how they are surviving. . . . I let some of my loans go at one point because I just couldn't afford to keep up the payments. I mean, things are a little better now, ten years after graduation, but they still aren't great. And I don't know what I would do if I was just starting out. . . . I mean with the debt, the changes in health care, the low salary . . . I can't imagine what it must be like. I thought I had it rough at first, but it is nothing compared to what these guys go through now.

Given this information, or the lack of it, one could wonder how a prospective student ends up choosing a particular chiropractic college. For some, who may have chiropractors in their families, the choices might be based on the recommendation of family members. In past decades, students often became involved in the profession because they had a relative, sometimes a parent, who was a chiropractor. Growing up with the ideology, attending chiropractic college is a natural progression into adulthood.

For others, it might have more to do with geographic region or the state the person is currently from or living. Some chiropractors think that newer graduates enter the profession because they could not get into medical school. This is a common assertion by some of the older chiropractors in the study, but in reality, many of the newer graduates were not interested in medical school, at least by their account. There appears to be a great desire to help people with injuries and illnesses, and generally speaking most of the chiropractors we interviewed were smart, kind, and compassionate, and had a passion to do something meaningful with their lives. That sense of purpose continues despite the buyers' remorse many feel about their experiences in chiropractic college. Jack offers this insight:

> I believe I make a difference with patients and I love what I do, but if I had to do it all over again? I think I would do something different. And I don't know anyone in this profession who would recommend it to their kids. In fact, I would discourage my kids from going into chiropractic, in part because of the costs and the low salary, but in part because it just feels like everyone is out for themselves—there's no sense of community, there's no sense of spirit de corps, there's just churning patients, struggling to make a living, and so many nut jobs out there making it hard for us to gain any credibility. And the colleges don't help by not being on the same page and taking advantage of students. To me they are just like the crazy doctors out there—taking their money, selling them things that will never happen, and not giving them very much in return.

Residency and Loan Forgiveness for Chiropractors

One of the things that many chiropractors discussed was the inadequacy of the training. Not only did they feel unprepared to launch a practice on their own, with many who did lamenting the mistakes they made. Several noted that, in retrospect, most of the mistakes were easily circumvented had their training included "tips and traps" made by others in the profession, but they also note the value and purpose in some type of residency program.

While some experts in the field have made the observation that graduates' experiences working as associates could be seen as a form of residency, others note that such a program could be a creative and profitable way for the Joint to expand its operation. Regardless of one's position on the issue, the fact remains that despite the clinical hours that give students some exposure to treating patients in real time, a residency program would be a valuable addition not only for those students but for the credibility of the profession itself.

Resistance, however, is likely to come from conservative chiropractors, who, as we have seen, are highly resistant to transforming chiropractic medicine to resemble the medical school experience and creating the perception that chiropractors should look, act, and be trained like physicians. Still, there are enough chiropractic college leaders who see a greater value in a residency program than the current practice of using associates. As Jay, a provost at one of the chiropractic colleges, points out, "if there was a real residency program, chiropractors would likely refrain from eating their young."

What he means by this, as was mentioned in a previous chapter, is that residency programs would likely end the existing practice of chiropractors hiring new graduates and exploiting them for the purpose of building their practice only to find themselves fired by the chiropractor, who takes over treating the new patients the graduate recruited. As for Jack, a chiropractor who thinks the idea of prescription drugs and allowing chiropractors to be first-line primary care providers are progressive strategies, this may be the explanation for why it has not already happened. He says the following:

> That's why you will see residency programs take a long time to develop. All those guys like the guy I worked for, who made me memorize scripts and grow his practice without any meaningful bonuses or profit sharing, won't have anyone to screw over. If grads are in a residency program, they may not need to work as an associate—maybe they will know enough about how to run a practice and not get exploited by some guy who only sees dollar signs.

Still, some programs are experimenting with educational experiences that could be seen as a form of residency programs for chiropractic students. Vinnie, a dean, offers what he is attempting to implement at his institution:

> The missing link at Northwestern was that students were hearing about all these things, but not really seeing anything in practice. So here at my institution, we do a clinic case conference, kind of like a grand rounds, where we discuss cases

and talk about clinical reasoning and then the students go and look for that in their offices . . . and at the same time they see how offices operate in the different dimensions and not just observe it but to come back and talk to us about it in those grand rounds. I hope the students say that all these experiences gave them a perspective on how they want to practice long before they are being asked to do it when they graduate. That's my hope anyway.

We're running parallel to the medical model, which has a residency program, which is an essential part of the overall education. In Switzerland, they have a mandatory two-year residency and the profession there is so much more respected than it is here. . . . It is so much more integrated with medicine. Med students and chiro students do the first two years together. . . . It is being copied in Denmark as well. There seems to be fear of residencies here and I think it's unfounded.

A lot of chiropractors whine and moan that in their first couple of years of practice they only made $35,000 or $ 40,000. But what do you think medical students get when they first start? The same thing. If we were to formalize that and admit to it they are junior doctors and have to basically pay the entry fee, as it were, but then we would see them in a different light. And the other part of what we're doing is that there is a lot of medical literature that says longitudinal clinical experience is so valuable rather than spotty drop-ins for surgery for a week, and psychiatry for a week, but some type of longitudinal experience is way more valuable. . . . So we're trying to give them a sixteen-week experience, and soon to be two eight-week experiences. They get to see over sixteen-weeks certain patients progress. . . . When you see a patient for the first time you don't get it right away in an in-depth kind of way.

Another issue for chiropractic colleges to address in particular is a student loan forgiveness program. Many mention the fact that they were told by their college advisors that if they worked in certain specialty categories, such as in rural areas or with particularly needy populations, such as veterans, a portion of their loans will be forgiven. This has been, until recently, a common way to attract providers to areas where there are shortages, be it teachers or medical personnel. However, this program, as many chiropractors later discovered, does not apply to chiropractic medicine. Jay explains the following:

So while I'm in school I'm beginning to see how much everything has cost me and I go to my advisor and say "Hey, what do I do about this?" She says, "Don't worry about it, you'll be fine." I'm like, "No, this is a lot of money and the fact that it is going to take me twenty-five years to pay it off matters a lot to me." She then tells me that there is a loan forgiveness program that all medical personnel are eligible for. I'm like, "Sweet, how do I sign up?" So she gives me a website and I file it away, thinking I'll go work in some rural area where they have a shortage of doctors and I'll be able to pare down some debt and then start my own practice. So I get near graduation and go searching on this website and can't find the information. So I call the Department of Education and they say,

> "No, you're not eligible for loan forgiveness." I'm like "What the hell? Was my advisor wrong, did they change the rules, what?" Either way, I'm screwed because now I have about a hundred and eighty grand in debt and no way to pay it down. I'm doing some work with the VA so that if they ever make us eligible for loan forgiveness I'll at least be able to say I did something for a while, but it's just another example of them [the chiropractic colleges] selling us snake oil.

Kathleen had this to say about loan forgiveness:

> The thing we don't have is, which a lot of other medical providers have is the public service loan forgiveness. There's another freakin' lie they told us in school, "Oh yeah, you're eligible for this," and I'm thinking, "Cool," and you get out and you're like, no we're not. But that's why I do stuff at the VA too because if anything every came up at the VA . . . I'd be eligible.

Joel points out that chiropractors make a community contribution similar to that of teachers who work in rural areas or those where there are severe shortages. He says the following:

> The other issue they brought up is the loan forgiveness part. . . . Many med schools are able to offer that chiropractors don't seem to get is a point of contention too . . . especially since the debt is about the same, especially if chiros can make the case that using chiropractic care is a great cost savings that would justify for some type of loan forgiveness. Not to mention, what we do in some communities is as much of a contribution to life there as what teachers do, but they get loan forgiveness if they work in rural area or with hard-to-reach populations. If we are willing to forego the earning potential of living in a city that might result in a more lucrative practice, why shouldn't we get some form of forgiveness? It's the same thing.

Given the enormous costs of attending, which in some cases exceed what medical students pay for their initial training, and given the salary differential, even accounting for a type of residency period, where physicians make in the $40,000 range, if the salary data is to be trusted, at-best chiropractors are going to make about what a physical therapist or physician assistant makes, somewhere in the $80,000 range.

However, this may be an overly optimistic assessment. As one franchise owner of the Joint pointed out, what he pays his chiropractors is what the market tolerates—and that is likely to be much less than the Department of Labor Statistics estimates. This trend is also underscored by the comments made by providers themselves about not making a lot of money in their own practices. Thus, it may be that some chiropractors would be incentivized to provide treatment to patients in needy areas if they could address some of the debt they carry after graduation.

The Council of Graduate Schools recently passed a resolution concerning the issue of graduate student debt and imploring Congress to modify the existing protocol on student loans for graduate students. Citing the fact that graduate study is qualitatively different from undergraduate education and the fact that most graduate students do not default on their loans, the primary source of funding for graduate study, the federal government needs to take the initiative and change the format in which student loans are managed (Council of Graduate Schools, 2017).

The need for adequate funding is critical, particularly for graduate students, who must rely on loans as their primary form of financial aid. Additionally, graduate students tend to have lower default rates and are considered by the Congressional Budget Office a good investment since they are more likely than other students to pay off their student loans (Council of Graduate Schools, 2017).

Historically, the interest rate for subsidized and unsubsidized student loans has been the same, whether fixed or variable. For PLUS loans, even with a higher interest rate and cap, the difference has been closer to 1.5 percent. However, in 2012, graduate students no longer qualified for the in-school interest subsidies. This means that graduate students are only eligible for unsubsidized loans and Grad PLUS loans which carry a higher interest rate and cannot be deferred. This puts graduate students in general, and minority students in particular, in a difficult situation, where the accumulated debt increases considerably. This is particularly true if graduate students carry debt from their undergraduate program of study (Council of Graduate Schools, 2017).

According to data drawn from the 2008 National Postsecondary Student Aid Study, the most recent data available, 73 percent of master's recipients had an average cumulative undergraduate and graduate debt of $41,000, and nearly two-thirds of those who received doctoral degrees had an average cumulative debt of $60,000. Minority graduate students, particularly African Americans, had cumulative averages higher than those of White students, with master's degree students averaging $52,000 and African-American doctoral students having an average cumulative debt of $68,000 (National Center for Educational Statistics, 2014). The proposal to eliminate the Grad PLUS program would further challenge graduate students' ability to pay for their programs and result in higher levels of debt as students would be forced to take out more private loans, which carry higher interest rates and restrictions.

Finally, the practice of income-based repayment of student loans (IBR), which was originally established for those students to repay their loans with a longer time frame than the traditional ten-year time limit, actually creates additional burdens for graduate students. IBR targeted those students who take on greater debt because of the costs of attending a graduate program of study at a time when the job market did not provide sufficient opportunities for graduates to obtain well-paying jobs. IBR allowed students to repay the loans over a longer period of time and forgives unpaid principal and interest after a specific period, such as twenty-five years. However, the student must pay federal and state taxes on what is owed as one-time taxable income (DeLise and Holt, 2012).

This tax provision substantially reduces the value of loan forgiveness, especially if the borrower is unable to pay the full tax liability in one year. For example, if a student has a loan that forgives $20,000, the student who receives loan forgiveness will have to pay $5,000 in additional income taxes the year the loan is forgiven. In addition, they would have to pay state income tax on that full amount as well. Depending on the state and its tax laws, that could result in an additional $1,400, assuming a flat 7 percent income tax. The combined cost to the student would be $6,400 the year the loan is forgiven. While it is still less than the full $20,000, it is not a true forgiveness program (DeLisle and Holt, 2012).

Melissa, who graduated last year, points out that the situation is so challenging, particularly since she is not eligible for the program as many of her colleagues were in the past. She says the following:

> Hey, I was told that if I paid my loans for like twenty-five years, then the loan would be forgiven. But in order to knock down any of the principal during that time, I have to pay like $2,500 a month just to stay current. That's a lot of money for me each month, so the idea of lasting like twenty-five years with debt like that, especially when I'm only making like $25,000 a year is tough. And I'm not sure what I'd make in a rural or underserved area, but geez, $25,000 is not a lot of money to begin with—think about it, I'm making like twelve bucks an hour for a forty-hour work week. And believe me, I'm likely working more than forty hours a week. Will that change and get better if I open my own practice? Maybe, but owning your own business doesn't mean you work less because you have all the responsibilities—you can't just show up, work and go home. So I may have to let my loans go for a while—I mean, seriously, I make less than $500 a week at my full time job. With $190,000 in loans, I have to take other jobs just to make the loan payment. Something is clearly wrong with this picture. And I had no idea until it was too late.

Melissa's lament is not an uncommon one heard by many providers during the study, including those who had been in the profession for three, five, ten, or even fifteen years. While some chiropractors said their financial situation improved somewhat, most still struggle with the burdens of their graduate college debt and many wonder if they will ever find a way beyond their current situation.

DISCUSSION

The sense of urgency felt by many segments within the profession has led to a rethinking of the role of the chiropractor in medicine, with the more integrative schools believing that if chiropractors were thought of as primary care physicians, the challenges relating to declining enrollments, salaries, credibility within the medical community, and professional standing for chiropractors will improve. This is a hotly contested issue, however, with many conservative chiropractors claiming that such a decision effectively eliminates the distinction of chiropractic medicine and risks the profession being engulfed by medicine in general.

Interestingly, as was seen in the last chapter, chiropractors often act inconsistently on core issues within the profession. On the one hand, chiropractors are adamant about their own autonomy and independence, claiming that they should not be regulated by outsiders. This has led to criticisms that chiropractors refuse to regulate the profession from providers who engage in dubious and even outright fraudulent practices for the sake of their own freedoms.

However, at the same time, chiropractors are quick to condemn organizations like the Joint as being unsafe, unfair, and a shady practice within the profession. Similarly, in this instance with regard to the training of chiropractic students, the chiropractic community criticizes its colleagues for having different philosophies of chiropractic colleges, but are unwilling to create a set of meaningful standards from which all colleges should operate.

Moreover, a common theme also appears to be that when one group or entity seems to be gaining any level of progress or success, such as the Joint with its success in attracting patients to their clinics or with chiropractic colleges that appear to gain some momentum in legitimizing the profession, the chiropractic community rallies against them with a concerted collective effort. While these efforts are admirable and somewhat effective at times, perhaps the community could consider marshaling such efforts in a positive way rather than in response to some type of threat from within. Instead of criticizing the Joint for its ability to find a niche within the market for chiropractic services, and doing so in an innovative way, perhaps the community could learn from such a model and adapt, as all businesses do in a free market system.

Similarly, instead of filing complaints against the accrediting body for certifying some chiropractic colleges for implementing a different philosophy, perhaps a collective effort could be created that begins a dialogue about finding a unified philosophy of treatment. If the profession were able to do this, then the chiropractic colleges would adapt to industry standards. Instead, we have an example of the horse driving the carriage, where chiropractic colleges are the catalysts behind changes to the profession.

While it is not clear that the integrative/Reformist approach to chiropractic medicine will succeed in creating a sense of legitimacy within the profession or to change the way the public perceives chiropractors, the realities are that the medical community will continue to perceive and portray chiropractors in a negative light until such time that they adopt a more empirical approach to what they do and the evidence indicates some level of success. Thus, the chiropractic colleges, who themselves operate independent of providers, must ensure viability by creating and implementing curricula that provide its students with the empirically proven techniques that foster the credibility the profession needs to survive in the future. The current model indicates that many students are not interested in accumulating significant amounts of debt for a salary that pays what a mid-level provider earns.

The consistently low enrollments should be an indicator that prospective students are not interested in a career as a chiropractor as in the past. Whether this means the profession and the colleges alter the landscape in an attempt to transform them into primary care physicians is not necessarily the answer. As many observers have noted, patients do not think of chiropractors as primary care providers and likely will not in the future.

As chiropractors cling to the idea of autonomous and independent medical providers, the realities of medicine, along with the changes in health care in the United States, will force them to conceptualize their self-perceptions with the realities of what role they can realistically play in medicine. Somewhere in that discussion, a transformation of the training they receive must occur, as it is unrealistic to expect students to continue to absorb hundreds of thousands of dollars in student loan debt for a profession that does not significantly return on that investment.

Such a position will likely be met with hostility and resistance, as it likely means chiropractors will have to adjust their understanding of the role they play, but that is already happening whether chiropractors want it to or not. This is a sobering development for chiropractic colleges, as they will likely be forced to move away from their current model to one that is more austere and simplified, with far less complexity and costs.

REFERENCES

Carnegie Foundation. 2014. *Carnegie Classification Systems*. Available at http://carnegieclassifications.iu.edu

Council of Graduate Schools. 2017. *The Future of Graduate Education Is the Future of America: A Call to Action*. Available at http://cgsnet.org/sites/default/files/CGS_Position_Statement_Student_Loan_Interest_Rates.pdf; see also Council of Graduate Schools, 2013. *Graduate Enrollments and Degrees, Fine and Field Report. 2002–2012*. Washington, DC: Council of Graduate Schools.

Delisle, J. and Holt, A. 2012. "Safety Net or Windfall: Examining Changes to Income-Based Repayment for Federal Loans." *New America Foundation.* Available at https://static.newamerica.org/attachments/2332-safety-net-or-windfall/NAF_Income_Based_Repayment.18c8a688f03c4c628b6063755ff5dbaa.pdf

Foundation for Vertebral Subluxation. 2012. "Chiropractic Colleges Not Preparing Graduates for Business Aspect of Practice." *The Chronicle of Chiropractic*, August 12th. Available at http://chiropractic.prosepoint.net/40840

National Board of Chiropractic Examiners, 2017. *Preparing for Exams.* Available at http://mynbce.org/prepare/spec

"Seventeen Statistics about Medical School Student Debt." 2017. *Becker's ASC Review.* Available at http://www.beckersasc.com/asc-turnarounds-ideas-to-improve-performance/17-statistics-about-medical-school-student-debt.html

U.S. Department of Education, National Center for Educational Statistics. 2014. *Trends in Student Financing of Graduate and First Professional Education, Selected Years 1995-6 to 2007-8.* Available at https://nces.ed.gov/pubs2011/2011217.pdf

———. 2017. *Fast Facts.* Available at https://nces.ed.gov/fastfacts/display.asp?id=40

———. 2017. *Integrated Postsecondary Education Data System.* Available at https://nces.ed.gov/ipeds/InsidePages/UseTheData?pageid=58

Chapter 7

Health Care Reform and Chiropractic Medicine

Being at the heart of this study and a central issue for all chiropractors and medical professionals, health care reform in the United States has significantly impacted life for virtually everyone involved in some aspect of medicine. In every interview and conversation about chiropractic care, the topic of concern inevitably led to an emotional discussion about the changes in health care and how they are adversely affecting the ability of chiropractors to sustain their practices and even the profession as a whole.

To be fair, the changing landscape of medicine and health care has transitioned away from the independent and autonomous profession it once was to one that is more responsive to the model of managed care, leaving physicians, and, in particular, chiropractors, facing a significantly different future than what many had perhaps expected. As health care continues to evolve in such a way that providers may be better suited to be employees of hospitals, or who find a particular niche in the marketplace that is not impacted by insurance coverage, the future of health care could render the chiropractic profession irrelevant, unnecessary, or marginalized like many primary care physicians.

For chiropractors in particular, who are seemingly steadfast in their desire to remain solo practitioners, unwilling to consolidate and collaborate into larger practices, the future direction of health care could render them a casualty of modern medicine. This may be one of the reasons why so many chiropractors and chiropractic colleges are advocating for a Reformist approach, where chiropractors could be seen as primary care providers. The alternative is that chiropractors may be relegated to providing a limited range of treatments and must compete with other professions who perform similar functions. However, as we have seen, the public and other health care practitioners do not think of chiropractors as primary care providers and there is some evidence that they are not trained to make an array of diagnoses. However, the shortage of primary care physicians, likely a result of the greater level of specialization in medicine, may create a window for chiropractors who have received additional training in primary care medicine.

Such a tactic is a risky one, however, because it is based on the premise that the medical field, and more importantly the insurance industry, will recognize and trust that chiropractors can and will meet the demand. Such a strategy also assumes that nurse practitioners and physician assistants will not be elevated to meet those needs with additional training. In such a situation, the gamble of revising the role of chiropractors as primary care providers may backfire.

Thus, the issues related to health care reform, for all of medicine in general and for chiropractors in particular, are complicated ones and the future of medicine is uncertain. As health care reform is perhaps one of the most pressing issues in American society today, a more thorough discussion is warranted. This chapter explores the idea of health care reform and offers insight into how and in what ways the existing and proposed changes could impact the chiropractic profession.

THE SPIRALING COSTS OF HEALTH CARE

The research points to a host of factors that influence health care reform in this country. Included in this discussion would be the explosive costs of health care, which includes fees charged by hospitals and physicians as well as the increased costs of medication. Related to this trend is the increased specialization of medicine, which emphasizes a particular focus that may or may not meet the needs of most citizens in this country. A third factor in the health care reform discussion involves the aging of the American population, which puts greater pressure on the existing health care infrastructure to absorb a larger patient load who have a variety of needs as a result of getting older (Alonso-Zaldivar, 2016).

There are also social factors at play, where people without health insurance who tend to be poor, have a variety of medical issues, and often use emergency rooms as their primary source of health care. Such a tactic increases the overall costs of providing care and reduces the continuity of care for patients. The development of medications to treat patients for a variety of illnesses has addressed part of the problem for the poor seeking treatment, but there have been dramatic increases in the cost of medications as well (Schumock et al., 2017).

Some experts contend that the current model is unsustainable and that the existing fee-for-services model will continue to increase costs to a point where very few will be able to pay unless the government is involved in health care (Nichols, 2017). Others point out that the single payer system, while popular in other countries, has not had a successful track record in the United States. As an example, critics of the single payer system point to the Veterans Administration (VA), where the problems with its infrastructure and ability to effectively treat patients is used as an illustration that the federal government is ill-equipped to handle such a large-scale endeavor (Waldman, 2014).

The Costs of Health Care in the United States

In 2016, a report issued by the Department of Health and Human Services (DHHS) showed that health care spending is growing at a faster rate than the national economy. Growth is expected to average about 5.8 percent from 2015 to 2025. National expenditures for health care were $3.35 trillion in 2016, which is approximately $10,345 for every man, woman, and child in the United States. These expenditures represented about 18 percent of the U.S. Gross Domestic Product (GDP) in 2015. The rise in health care costs is expected to increase to 20 percent of the economy by 2025. The distribution of the $3.35 trillion in health care costs consists of hospitals, which account for about a third of the costs; doctors and other providers account for another 20 percent, and prescription drugs bought through pharmacies comprise another 10 percent (Alonso-Zaldivar, 2016).

These costs are extraordinary: where health care spending per capita in the United States is more than double that of other developed countries. Yet, the health outcomes from this additional spending show results that are no better than peer countries—and in some cases they are worse. Part of the reason for these poor results is incompetence, greed, and waste. The Institute of Medicine, for example, has estimated that about 30 percent of total health care spending goes to unnecessary, ineffective, overpriced, and wasteful services. This cost, more nearly $800 billion, is more than the entire budget for K–12 education (Peterson Foundation, 2017).

The DHHS report showed that spending on prescription drugs also grew significantly. According to the Centers for Medicare and Medicaid Services (CMS), retail drug spending increased about 13 percent in 2014 to nearly $300 billion and another 9 percent in 2015 to nearly $325 billion. These increases far exceeded any other rate of growth in health care and account for about 10 percent of the total health care spending.

Efforts to curb the costs of prescription drugs have not had their intended effect. As an illustration, the dramatic costs in drugs such as epinephrine auto injectors, also known as the EpiPen, garnered considerable negative publicity when the manufacturer increased the cost from about $57 in 2007 to $615.58 in 2016. Since 2007, when Mylan Corporation took control of the drug, there has been a steady increase in the price—and it is the only drug of its kind on the market. The actual costs of the drug are about a dollar per device and children who need the EpiPen are advised to have at least two, one in the home and one that is accessible at all times.

In response, corporate executives cite product improvements as the justification for the increased costs, but little in the way of actual improvements have been documented (Woodyard and Layton, 2016). While Myaln's CEO took considerable criticism for this action, the EpiPen is not the only drug on the market that saw skyrocketing costs. Turing Pharmaceuticals raised the price of one of its drugs, Daraprim, from $13 to over $750 per tablet. Despite pressure from the media, there is no indication that this trend will subside any time soon (Schumock et al., 2017).

The Specialization of Medicine

As was mentioned, a sizable portion of the costs of health care involves physician fees. These fees are often the result of the need for patients to see a specialist for the particular problem they are experiencing. But overspecialization in medicine is a problem as well. As more and more medical students choose to specialize in a particular area, it reduces the number of general and family practitioners, who see patients for a variety of illnesses and make recommendations to specialists for certain types of care. There are many good reasons for specialization in medicine, particularly in developing a sense of expertise in a refined area, but managed care requires a referral from a primary care physician.

As information and technology improve society's ability to diagnose and treat illnesses, the body of knowledge expands, making it quite challenging to stay abreast of all the changes. Specialization reduces some of that burden by allowing practitioners to refine their skill and knowledge base and to actually become better at treating patients than they would otherwise. Specialization also allows for physicians to earn more by developing this level of expertise and reduce the administrative responsibilities as it relates to billing for insurance.

For example, consider the average salaries of the top and bottom five areas in medicine in Table 7.1 (Hamblin, 2015).

The salaries commanded by these specialties are driven by the fees they can charge patients and insurance companies for their services. While some of these physicians are primarily engaged in research, particularly those in the bottom ranking, family medicine, which represents the entry point for most patients into the medical system in the United States, pays substantially less than virtually every other treatment-providing physician. This degree of specialization continues to reshape medicine and its practice. There are currently 24 specialty boards related to the AMA that certify physicians to practice nearly 150 specialties (Fromson, 2011). There are many reasons

Table 7.1 Top and Bottom Five 2015 Average U.S. Physician Salaries by Specialty

Top Five	
Neurosurgery	$609,639
Orthopedic Surgery	$535,668
Thoracic Surgery	$471,137
Cardiology	$436,849
Vascular Surgery	$428,944
Bottom Five	
Pediatric Endocrinology	$157,394
Pediatric Infectious Diseases	$163,658
Pediatric Nephrology	$183,730
Pediatrics	$205,610
Endocrinology	$217,610
Family Medicine	$227,541

why a medical student might choose a particular area of specialty, including prestige, salary, working hours, and so on.

At the same time, however, with more specialties comes a shortage of primary care physicians, which creates a backlog of patients who need a referral to see a specialist. It also results in hospital emergency rooms becoming the de facto primary care center for some people, particularly those who do not have any other access to medical care. This is the most expensive way to treat patients, thereby contributing to the escalating costs of health care, and it results in a lower continuity of care for the patient, since they see whichever provider is on duty, who may not have a comprehensive history of the patient's health.

But the problem does not end with the shortage of primary care physicians or the high salaries of specialists. Even within the profession, there is competition among subspecialties or even within practices in the same area of expertise. As Fromson (2011) points out, the shortage of specialists has generated numerous strategies to entice students nearing the end of their training—including salaries that are $100,000 higher than they were just a few years earlier, extravagant signing bonuses, paid living expenses, payment of student loans, very convenient work schedules, which include extensive vacation time, and no obligation for taking call or working weekends.

In 2010, the Association of American Medical College's Center for Workforce Studies predicted that there would be a shortage of nearly 45,000 primary care physicians and 62,000 non-primary care specialists by 2020 (Fromson, 2011). If some of the extraordinary offers that are described in Fromson's (2011) article are any indication, it appears that the prediction of the physician shortages is already being seen.

Thus, the specialization of medicine is creating pressure on hospitals and medical practices, which contribute to the continuing costs of medicine, while at the same time creating a shortage of primary care physicians. The end result is a limited access to care, longer wait times to receive it, and the use of other alternatives to meet patient needs.

Longevity and the Aging of America

The 2016 DHHS report showed that Medicare and Medicaid are expected to grow more rapidly than private insurance as the population ages. In fact, by 2025, the government will account for 47 percent of all health care spending. Such a startling prediction indicates that we may end up with a single payer system simply as a result of the Baby Boom generation aging and the government paying the costs of their health care. But even the larger numbers of people being eligible for care do not tell the entire story. The DHHS estimates that about 5 percent of the population account for nearly half of the health care spending in a given year. This means that even with affordable health care for everyone, its use will remain significantly uneven.[1]

However, not everyone believes that the aging population contributes greatly to the escalating health care costs. In 2013 a report released by the Society of Actuaries, using data from the Health Care Cost Institute, examined the impact of aging on health care costs. The study, entitled *Health Care Costs from Birth to Death*, showed that the average fifty-five-year-old retiree will spend almost a quarter of a million dollars more on health care than a person retiring at the age of sixty-five, assuming they both live to the age of eighty-five. The study also showed that America's aging population is not an overwhelming factor in the discussion of increased health care spending, although the cost of children's health care is increasing. Health care costs are twice as high for people with cancer, circulatory, or musculoskeletal conditions than for those people without them. The report also showed that the aging population in this country has consistently contributed an average increase of less than one half of 1 percent per year to health care costs for over a decade.

While the study should prompt one to pause and consider the actual impact of the aging population on health care costs, there can be little doubt that as the population gets older and there are greater demands for treatment, those costs will continue to escalate, which will then be passed along to taxpayers.

THE HISTORY OF HEALTH CARE IN AMERICAN

From the outset, it appears that the medical community has generally opposed any legislation that curbed the autonomy and authority of physicians. Even in its earliest forms, such as when Harry Truman first proposed a national health insurance program for all Americans in 1945, the AMA argued that such a program would be a form of socialism and voiced its opposition to it. More than likely, such a move was not based on political ideology, in that the AMA was against socialism per se; rather the issue really focused on who should be making decisions about health care in this country (Updegrove, 2012).

Traditionally, physicians have felt that they were in the best position to not only treat patients but to decide on matters of policy and what types of programs were needed. Truman's efforts were perhaps one of the first real threats to medicine and its control over health care. Generally speaking, the medical profession has been opposed to programs like worker's compensation, Social Security, and voluntary health insurance. They have also strongly opposed any proposal for national health insurance. In fact, Truman's plan died in Congress, largely because of the opposition from the AMA (Updegrove, 2012; Cockerham, 2017).

In the 1970s President Nixon attempted to elevate the national conversation about health insurance that was tied to the concept of Health Management Organizations. However, the Watergate scandal, and Nixon's involvement in it, derailed any further discussion about a national health insurance program. The scandal also resulted in Nixon's resignation from office. President Jimmy Carter also called attention to the need for national health insurance during his first term, but his failure to rescue the hostages from Iran ended the discussion of health insurance (Brinkley, 1998).

Like his predecessors, in 1994, President Clinton attempted to tackle the thorny problem of health care and national health insurance. As it had been the case for generations, the problems of rising costs and the number of people who were without health insurance pushed the issue to the national spotlight. At the time, there was some optimism that Clinton's plan would succeed. However, when the plan was delivered to Congress in 1993, numerous lobby groups attempted to delay or derail it. The small-business lobby was strongly opposed because it would have required businesses with only a few employees to pay most (80 percent) of the health insurance for their workers (Riley, 2017).

The AMA continued to oppose governmental control over health care delivery and the potential loss of income for doctors, drug companies, and hospitals. Insurance companies opposed it because of the price controls, while labor unions and the elderly opposed it on the basis of caps on health benefits that their plans already contained. Add this to the lack of consensus between Democrats and Republicans, a common feature on an issue like health care reform, and the plan was destined for failure (Moffitt, 1993).

In 1994, President Clinton vowed to take up the issue again in the next year, but his sex scandal and impeachment trial derailed any further discussion of health care reform. However, the Clinton plan had two important features. It not only made health care reform a central issue for the general public, but also prompted a massive reorganization of American health care into a delivery system that resulted in what is now known as managed care (Moffitt, 1993; Riley, 2017).

President Johnson's Contribution to Health Care: Medicare and Medicaid

President Johnson was the only president before Obama to have any meaningful success with limited health care reform by establishing Medicare and Medicaid in 1965 (Updegrove, 2012; Cockerham, 2017). It was during the 1960s that evidence revealed private health insurance was limited in its success, particularly in meeting the needs of the poor and the elderly. While some of the reasons behind Johnson's success had to do with timing and the composition of Congress, another factor was the realization by many experts that the AMA could not always be relied upon to put the public's interests regarding health care above its own.

During this period the AMA claimed that "physicians cared for the elderly" and "knew their health needs better than anyone else." Officials of the AMA also commented on the fact that federal health insurance was incompatible with "good" medicine. These comments came as a result of continued evidence that the needs of the elderly were not being adequately met by physicians and part of the reason had to do with costs (Updegrove, 2012).

Unlike previous efforts, where the AMA played a key role in the failure of health care legislation, Congress passed the Medicare and Medicaid amendments of the Social Security Act of 1965. This was considered by many experts to be a watershed event in the history of politics, as it represented the first time that Congress played a key role in health care policy and that the AMA was no longer the sole domain of organized medicine. As we will see, this decision has played a pivotal role in how medicine has been understood since then (Updegrove, 2012).

Medicare, which differs from Medicaid, in that the former provides medical and hospital insurance for people aged sixty-five and older regardless of their financial resources. It also includes people under the age of sixty-five who receive cash benefits from Social Security. There are specific deductibles and coinsurance payments for which the beneficiary is responsible, as well as overall limits to the program, but most of the cost is absorbed by the federal government. Hospital insurance is covered through Social Security deductions and does not require a monthly premium if the recipient paid Medicare taxes during their working lifetime (Cockerham, 2017).

The medical insurance plan, which is voluntary, is paid by participants and the cost depends upon the plan selected from those available in a given state. In 2006, prescription drug coverage was made available to everyone with Medicare and currently there are a wide range of plans with a corresponding monthly fee. People living below the federal poverty line or just above it, do not have to pay these costs, and low-income retirees pay according to a sliding scale (Cockerham, 2017).

Oversight of the Medicare program is provided by the U.S. Department of Health and Human Services, and is supervised by the Bureau of Health Insurance of the Social Security Administration. However, most of the actual operation of reimbursements and payments are handled by commercial insurance companies and Blue Cross/Blue Shield plans that review claims and make payments. In 2014, a total of $597 billion in Medicare benefits was paid to fifty-five million people aged sixty-five and older and disabled people, which represented about 14 percent of the federal budget. The projected spending according to the Congressional Budget Office is $1.2 trillion by 2024 (Kaiser Family Foundation, 2015).

Medicaid involves the federal government sharing in the payments made by state welfare agencies to health care providers for services to the poor. Medicaid essentially gives the states federal matching funds, ranging from 50 to 76 percent of expenditures, depending on the per capita income of the states involved. Each state is required to cover all needy persons receiving cash assistance. States are allowed to include not only the financially needy but also the aged, the blind, and the disabled poor as well as their dependent children and families. In 1986 Congress extended Medicaid coverage to children under five years of age and pregnant women with incomes below the federal poverty level. Medicaid was expanded under the Affordable Care Act to cover people low-income persons earning 133 percent of the poverty line (National Conference of State Legislatures, 2017).

However, in 2012 the U.S. Supreme Court ruled that states could opt out of the Medicaid expansion and as of 2016, nineteen states had done so. When the percentage of the U.S. population covered by Medicaid and Medicare is combined, along with those covered under children's health insurance plan or CHIP, approximately 40 percent of all Americans in 2016 had all or most of their health insurance needs paid for by federal and state governments (Cockerham, 2017).

The upshot of this involvement by the federal government in matters of health care essentially eliminates the question of whether they should or should not be involved in health care. The real question, then, is to what extent is the federal government going to be involved in health care and providing coverage for citizens.

Managed Care in Medicine: A Game Changer

As was mentioned, President Clinton's legacy relating to health care in this country relates to the development of managed care, a process which altered how medicine was delivered that continues today. The previous model had been an office-based, fee-for-services system, however, Managed care emerged as a result of businesses and industry attempting to control escalating health care costs for its workers. Managed care is the term used to describe how health organizations, such as Health Management Organizations (HMOs) or PPOs (Private Payer Organizations) "manage" or control the costs of health care by supervising and monitoring the work of doctors, hospitals and the like, as well as limiting visits to specialists to a particular managed care network and requiring prior authorization for hospitalization. It has become, in effect, the most common form of health care delivery in this country (Cockerham, 2017).

Thus, managed care brings a third party into the interaction between physicians and patients, someone who is paying more attention to the bottom line and by extension, the decision making process. The idea is that there is an outside party, the insurance company, who sees to it that the care provided by the physician is reasonable and the least costly alternative. To discourage inefficient and unnecessary treatment, *capitation financing* was introduced. This is a fixed monthly amount paid by the employee and the employer and in exchange the health care provider offers care for the person and their family at little or no cost. Obviously, given the costs of health care, it is in the best interest of that health care provider to be cost-effective with the treatment it provides (Cockerham, 2017).

Primary care providers are designed to be the gatekeepers in this system by limiting the use of referrals to specialists. Patients are also required to see primary care physicians that are a part of the insurance carrier's network and are discouraged from going outside that circle of providers. This system is said to be more efficient and serves to contain some of the rising costs involved in the delivery of health care. The process began with the federal government and the creation of *diagnosis-related groups*, known more commonly as *DRGs*. These were used to classify patients based on their diagnosis, how much and the type of care they received, in an effort to standardize the reimbursement given to health care providers for treating patients (Davis, 2017). However, hospitals responded by seeking to shift costs from government payers to private payers (insurance companies).

In turn, insurance companies, in an attempt to address the outcry from business and industry about escalating costs, turned to a managed care system. In doing so, the historical autonomy afforded to doctors, who dominated medicine and medical treatments, transitioned into a model with a form of accountability that is focused on outcome measures and standardized criteria for treatment. Managed care forced physicians to be accountable to those who had to pay the bill: insurance companies, the federal government, and employers. In the process, managed care became a business much like any other, where controlling costs and market sensitivity drove decision making. This model theoretically spelled the end of doctors making all of the decisions in terms of patient care and health care policy.

So has it worked? Has managed care controlled costs and made a positive impact on health care reform? The data suggests that initially costs were contained, but lately that trend has changed. Between 1993 and 1997 health care's portion of the GDP was about 13.5 percent. In 1995 the U.S. Department of Commerce estimated that health care costs would exceed 15 percent of the GDP. Until 2006, the percentage hovered around the 13.5 percent mark. However, in 2007, the costs jumped to 16.2 percent and steadily rose to 17.4 percent in 2014. In 2016, it reached 17.8 percent and the total cost of health care in the United States has reached $3.25 trillion (Peterson Foundation, 2017).

Some of the reasons for this increase may have been a result of dissatisfaction with managed care by consumers. Americans, by and large, are interested in choice and the freedom to select their preferred provider. As managed care evolved, with more insurance companies authorizing more referrals to specialists, costs to patients increased.

While the initial decreases may have been a result of certain efficiencies and restrictions of care, experts are now cautiously assessing managed care as a moderate success, but even this may be an unfair assessment since the costs could not be known had it not been implemented, and there is no reason to believe that physicians would have self-imposed cost constraints nor could the impact of such a decision be calculated. Thus, it may be unfair to criticize managed care from this vantage point because it might have been a lot worse without it.

Aside from the economic costs related to managed care are the social and cultural costs to medicine. As managed care changes the medical landscape, the role of physicians has changed as well. As they become less autonomous and more like employees working for hospitals, along with the prescription-laden way medicine is practiced, many physicians have expressed dissatisfaction with the profession and medicine in general. However, given the costs and administrative challenges to operating and managing a private practice, many physicians have become accustomed to the idea of the loss of autonomy. As a result of managed care and the changing way medicine is practiced, job satisfaction among physicians has become an issue, particularly with primary care physicians and general practitioners (Rabin 2014; Adams, 2012; Punke, 2013).

The realities of health care costs have resulted in efforts by some states to create and implement their own health insurance plans for its citizens, especially the poor. However, the scope of this problem is so large and the costs so extraordinary, despite limited success in places like Massachusetts, Hawaii, and Vermont, most states are unable to resolve the issue. However, there is a growing body of evidence that shows people who have health insurance end up living longer and in better health than those who do not. It is this persistent finding that has led to so many efforts to reform health care in this country and it was also the impetus for the Affordable Care Act, also known as Obamacare.

The Affordable Care Act/Obamacare

With the election of President Obama in 2009, along with Democrats controlling both the House and the Senate, a power shift occurred that pushed health care to the forefront of public policy. Obama put health care reform at the top of the domestic agenda at a time when the country was experiencing a major recession. Despite this economic upheaval, along with the wars in Iraq and Afghanistan, Republicans strongly opposed health care reform. Concerns were raised about rising health care costs, the ability of the government to operate and manage health care systems, along with concerns about the need for cuts in Medicare benefits.

The health care reform bill, officially called the Patient Protection and Affordable Care Act, also known as Obamacare, was passed in March 2010. Important elements of this legislation include the following:

1. The elimination of denying coverage to patients for preexisting conditions;
2. Minimum level of benefits, determined by the federal government, would be required of all health insurance plans;
3. State insurance exchanges were created so that a wide range of health insurance plans can be offered at competitive prices;
4. People who are not covered by health insurance through their employer can purchase coverage through state exchanges;
5. People under the age of sixty-five who already have health insurance can purchase plans from the exchanges and who earn up to four times the federal poverty line will receive government subsidies to help pay the cost;
6. Low-income people under the age of sixty-five earning below 133 percent of the poverty line will be covered by an expanded Medicaid program;
7. Small businesses can buy insurance for their employees through the exchanges and get tax credits.
8. Children can remain on their parents' health insurance plan until the age of twenty-six;

9. People would generally be required to purchase health insurance or pay a penalty added to their federal income tax. Some groups are exempt from this rule, such as Native Americans, religious objectors, and people with hardships. Additionally, employers who have more than fifty employees who do not provide health insurance coverage pay a penalty. Penalties for individuals can be less than $100 or more than $1,000, depending on their income and were scheduled to increase in future years (Cockerham, 2017).

The cost for such a plan was estimated by the Congressional Budget Office to be approximately $1.1 trillion over the next decade. About half of these costs were said to be covered by spending cuts and limits on Medicare payments and other savings, while the other half was expected to come from higher Medicare taxes, fees and new taxes on drug manufacturers and others, along with penalties paid by businesses and uninsured individuals.

The ACA had several problems. For instance, initially the website for signing up for the insurance was not operational and it was difficult for some states to offer coverage until it had been fixed. Because individuals would be assessed a penalty if they did not sign up for health coverage, Obama was forced to waive the first year's penalties and extend the deadline for enrollment. When Obama did this without Congressional approval, Republicans in the House of Representatives filed a lawsuit charging the he had changed a federal law without Congress's approval (Schencker, 2014).

Second, despite President Obama's promise that people would be allowed to keep the insurance coverage they already had, many individuals and families had their policies cancelled or were required to pay higher prices for new ones. The new plans included provisions that some people did not need or want—such as paying for prenatal care for women past childbearing age. The health plans also had very high deductibles: over half of the plans had deductibles of $3,000 or more (Schencker, 2014).

In response, Obama allowed insurance companies to let people keep their old policies for another year, but some companies declined to do so because of the cost of issuing new policies with old benefits. Despite these challenges, as of 2016 about twenty million people enrolled in ACA health plans. However, a number of large health insurance providers ended their participation in state exchanges because of significant financial losses. The problem was further complicated by insurance companies raising the premiums for most existing plans. On average, ACA insurance premiums rose about 22 percent in 2016. While about 80 percent of people with ACA coverage received federal subsidies, nearly $33 billion, the other 20 percent of customers, had to pay the full amount of those increases (Cox, Claxton and Levitt, 2015).

Recall the stipulations of the ACA and the mandate for individuals to obtain health insurance and for employers to provide it for their employees or pay a fine. As a result of these and other questions, several lawsuits were filed against such mandates. Some states argued that it was unconstitutional to require people to purchase health insurance, similar to being forced to buy any commercial good or service as a condition of residency in the United States. Other issues focused on religious exemptions as well as forcing employers to purchase health insurance for their workers (Spakovsky, 2015).

The federal courts were inconsistent in their decisions on the constitutionality issue. In 2010, federal courts in both Virginia and Michigan found that the requirement to purchase health insurance was in fact constitutional, but another court in Virginia ruled that it was not. The argument in favor of the requirement asserted that the Commerce Clause of the Constitution allows Congress to oversee events and activities that impact interstate commerce. The federal government also argued that, because non-compliance with the law resulted in an income tax penalty, Congress was allowed to require health insurance based on its powers to tax citizens (Cockerham, 2017). The case was appealed to the U.S. Supreme Court and in *National Federation of Independent Small Businesses v. Sibelius* 576 U. S. _____ (2012), in a 5-4 vote, the Court agreed with the federal government. It also ruled that the expansion of Medicaid was legal but that Congress could not coerce states into participating by withholding existing Medicaid payments. The states were given the option of opting out of expanding their Medicaid programs (Liptak, 2012).

The Supreme Court also addressed the religious exemption and employer requirement issues. In *Little Sisters of the Poor v. Burwell*, 578 U. S. _____ (2016), Roman Catholic nuns had sought an injunction requiring them to provide contraceptive devices to their employees at a convent because it violated their religious beliefs. In a second case, *Hobby Lobby Stores v. Burwell* 568 U. S. _____ (2012), a family-owned business run on religious principles wanted an exception from having to pay for contraceptive devices as outlined in the ACA. The Supreme Court ruled in favor of the plaintiffs in these cases, granting the injunction by the Roman Catholic nuns and exempting Hobby Lobby from paying for contraceptive services of its employees.

The GOP Alternative to Obamacare

With the presidential election expected to take place in 2016, questions remained about the ACA. Hilary Clinton was expected to win the race, thereby preserving Obamacare and its parameters. In fact, the media calculated that Clinton had an 85 to 91 percent chance of winning the presidency; however, the actual outcome was quite different. The Republican candidate, Donald Trump, was elected to the presidency and Republicans had the majority in both the House and the Senate (Who Will Win the Presidency?, 2016).

Trump went on the record early in his candidacy that he would repeal the ACA and replace it with a better health plan. He also stated that health care reform was one of his top priorities if elected. Despite the fact that millions of people would be left without coverage with a repeal of Obamacare, Trump promised that people would not lose coverage when the ACA was repealed. Trump stated he would likely keep some of the provisions of the ACA, such as requiring insurers to cover people with preexisting conditions and allowing parents to keep their children on their policies until they are twenty-six years old (Laszewski, 2016).

Trump also said that he felt that there should be an end to the Medicaid expansion, eliminating the subsidies to the middle class, and ending both the tax penalties for not having health insurance and the taxes created to help pay the cost of the ACA. Trump also stated that the single payer model that was proposed by the Democrats, referred to as "Medicare for all" would be eliminated. While Trump began to follow through on his promise in his first days in office, the Republican party began crafting their own version of the ACA (Lawzewski, 2016).

A significant effort by Senate Republicans to pass health care legislation collapsed in the July of 2017 when, after months of discussion and debate, Republican John McCain of Arizona, joined by two of his colleagues, Senators Susan Collins of Maine and Lisa Murkowski of Alaska, voted to stop a revised and limited version of an Obamacare repeal bill. The "skinny" repeal, as it has been called, was defeated 49–51, falling just short of the fifty votes needed to advance it (Parks, Rogin, Parkinson and Caplan, 2017).

Trump's Alternative Plan to Kill Obamacare

On July 28, 2017, President Trump threatened to end government payments to health insurers if Congress did not pass a new health care bill. In a Twitter message, President Trump said, "if a new HealthCare Bill is not approved quickly, BAILOUTS for Insurance Companies and BAILOUTS for members of Congress will end very soon!" This tweet occurred just after the Senate failed to repeal parts of the Affordable Care Act. Trump referenced the bailouts, which amount to approximately $8 billion in subsidies the federal government pays to insurers to lower the price of health coverage for some Americans. The threat to suspend these payments, which are determined by the U. S. Department of Health and Human Services, is questionable and will likely result in legal action by the insurance companies, since there remain real questions about whether the language of Obamacare authorized the payments (Kessler, 2017).

Republicans have questioned the legality of the payment of subsidies to insurance companies since at least 2014. The ACA provides two types of subsidies to help low- and middle-income people pay for insurance on the exchanges. Premium subsidies defray the cost of premiums for people making less than four times the poverty level. For those who make even less, cost-sharing reductions help cover the costs of deductibles and other out-of-pocket expenses (Zernike, 2017).

Although similar in some ways, the premium subsidies are refundable tax credits that go to individuals. For cost-sharing reductions, the ACA requires insurers to cut their lowest income customers a deal on expenses. The statute says the federal government will reimburse insurers for doing so. The crux of the matter is that the Constitution states that "no money shall be drawn from the Treasury, but in Consequence of Appropriations made by law." This means that it is not enough for a law to state that the government will make a payment for something, Congress must adopt a law that specifically appropriates the money to make that payment. While the ACA does link the premium subsidies to an existing appropriation, it does not say anything about cost-sharing reductions. This is the legal dispute Republicans called attention to in the lawsuit (Zernike, 2017).

Initially, the lawsuit was seen as political maneuvering—Republicans lost the battle and so they were trying to gain some type of victory any way they could. To be fair, House Republicans had a point—while federal courts had never really been involved in the resolution of an appropriations bill—something Congress and the Executive branch typically worked out in the past to reach a reasonable compromise—that did not happen in this particular case (Bagley, 2017).

The Obama administration identified the appropriations problem before the exchanges were launched and went to Congress to request cost-sharing funds. Congress refused and the administration made the legal argument that the appropriation for the premium subsidies could serve in the same capacity for the cost-sharing reductions. Both types of subsidies serve the same purpose, so the administration argued that Congress must have intended the same appropriation to serve for both types of subsidies (Bagley, 2017).

A district court judge ruled that the House of Representatives had a solid argument and in May 2016, the court issued an opinion that the cost-sharing payments were unconstitutional and ordered them stopped. The district court delayed its injunction however to give the government time to appeal. Shortly after the appeal was filed by the Obama administration, Trump won the election. With the election of President Trump, the House asked the appeals court to put the case on hold because of the likely changes in health care policy that were forthcoming. The appeals court agreed to do so and ordered status reports every ninety days (Bagley, 2017).

It seemed evident from the Republican alternative to Obamacare, the American Health Care Act, that they wanted to eliminate the cost-sharing subsidies by 2020. By most accounts, if the Act had passed, Congress would have likely funded the cost-sharing payments during the transition period. However, that did not occur and the case has become a backdoor answer to the failed repeal of Obamacare (Bagley, 2017).

In sum, Republicans argue that Obamacare did not specify a source of funding for the program, making it illegal for the Department of Health and Human Services to distribute payments unless authorized by Congress (Washington Free Beacon, 2017). A pending court case, *House v. Price*, a lawsuit brought by Republican House of Representatives to sue the Obama administration, accused it of making billions of dollars in illegal cost-sharing payments to insurance companies (Bagley, 2017).

The threat to end the subsidies was one way that Trump could leverage an end to Obamacare without legislation, since it would result in companies raising premiums in the marketplace or stop offering coverage all together. Estimates by the Congressional Budget Office indicate that premiums would increase approximately 20 percent if the payments are not made (Newsline, 2017).

By summer 2017, many insurance companies had already withdrawn from the Obamacare markets after sustaining losses and express concern over the future of Obamacare as a reason for increasing premiums (Bloomberg, 2017). Predictions about the plan, including lingering uncertainty over the legality of the payments coupled with Trump's unreliability in decision making, led many experts to be concerned about insurers deciding not to take the chance by participating at all (Bagley, 2017; Bryan, 2017a).

On August 2, 2017, a federal court ruled that the President is not the only one with legal standing in this appeal. Should he decide to withdraw his appeal and allow the lower court injunction to stand, the latest court ruling indicates that all seventeen states and Washington, DC could intervene and continue the appeal. The court stated: "The states have filed within a reasonable time from when their doubts about adequate representation arose due to accumulating public statements by high-level officials both about a potential change in position and the Department's joinder with the House in an effort to terminate the appeal." (Bryan, 2017:12).

This changed the political leverage President Trump may have had in forcing Democrats to come to some sort of compromise on Obamacare in general and the proposed Trump care plan. What is not known is whether Trump will withdraw his appeal in an effort to force the issue of appropriations. This essentially puts the health care discussion to rest for a time, since Trump's leverage in Congress is dissipated and he can no longer force the issue of withholding payments. Despite his claim to continue the battle to repeal Obamacare, and despite his criticisms of Republicans in Congress, the reality is that Trump will likely have to let the health care issue rest until at least after the November 2017 elections.

This is a wise decision, particularly given that most Americans think Republicans in Congress should work on a new health care bill. According to a Reuters/Ipsos poll, 64 percent of people surveyed said they wanted to keep Obamacare either "entirely as is" or after fixing "problem areas." (Schectman, 2017). Thus, it appears that Obamacare will remain at the forefront of the health care policy for the foreseeable future.

OBAMACARE AND CHIROPRACTORS

Like many physicians, Obamacare has negatively impacted how chiropractors operate. In fact, public and private insurance have begun to reexamine how it reimburses all forms of medical treatment, but it also began paying closer attention to chiropractors than in the past. In general, while most plans vary somewhat, chiropractic care is limited to a specific number of treatments for a given problem, and it will not cover what is known as *maintenance care.* The reimbursement rates for chiropractic treatments have also been reduced: the average Medicare payment per adjustment is less than $25 (O'Donnell, Hoyer, and Alcindor, 2014). As one might imagine, this has had a significant impact on chiropractors and their ability to treat patients. One issue that commonly arises is the awkwardness of telling a patient when they have met their insurance plan's limit for the number of treatments. Steven talks about this and how it affects his practice. He says the following:

> Listen, the insurance company tells me that this patient only gets twelve adjustments per year. Now I'll tell you, if a patient comes in to see me for an injury, twelve visits is plenty. I shouldn't say this because my colleagues will scream at me, but twelve visits is a lot of visits. If I can't fix that patient's problem in twelve visits, then I'm either doing something wrong, I don't know what's going on, or I'm just trying to make money off that patient. But the problem starts when that patient is taken care of, they go back to work or doing whatever they were doing, and then they injure themselves again. Then they come back to me and in my mind, I start all over again, because that is a new injury. It's not the same problem, because I took care of that. But it's a new one. . . . It could even be an overuse injury, but it's new. So in my mind I should have another twelve or ten visits, or whatever the plan calls for. But then I usually get a call because I've seen this patient more than a dozen times and they go "Hey, what are you doing with this patient?" And when I try to tell them it is a new injury, they are skeptical and think I'm trying to milk them or something. I tell them "Look at my notes, look at the dates." But a lot of times they give me grief about it.

The issue of the maintenance care is a controversial one and continues to plague the profession. As was mentioned in a previous chapter, there are those providers who steadfastly believe that regular adjustments are a key to a patient's overall health, even if they do not subscribe to the traditional views of chiropractic, including the Innate. Rather, like brushing one's teeth, these providers believe they are preventing injuries and illnesses from occurring by having patients regularly adjusted. The problem is that insurance companies do not see these types of treatment the same way.

Another challenge with insurance companies relates to reimbursements. As Doug points out, in the past, insurance companies would provide a greater percentage of reimbursement for treatment than they do under Obamacare. He says the following:

> It used to be you'd get all you billed for—now? Sometimes I wonder if it is even worth the paperwork to get the $28 for an adjustment, especially since you have to call them up, fight with them over whether it was a legitimate treatment or medically necessary. And then you have to send over the documentation, then they may or may not approve it. Then next month, you have to do it all over again. It's crazy.

The general feeling by many chiropractors is that insurance companies, in an effort to cut costs, changed their view of chiropractic care as medically necessary. While this is a critical term used in the industry to justify treatment, some chiropractors think insurance companies see it as a way to cut corners. As Jim points out,

> Oh, I absolutely think insurance companies are seeing it differently. Nowadays, insurance companies are looking at chiropractic treatments as a luxury item that they can just eliminate among the many things they are cutting out of plans. So I end up having to use that term over and over again. . . . It's medically necessary, it's medically necessary. That's the only way they'll pay and it's because they don't want to get sued. But insurance companies are doing everything they can to shortchange their customers and refusing to pay for chiropractic services is just another example.

Another area that troubles some chiropractors is being the one who informs the patient of his or her insurance limits. This puts them in the awkward position of telling a patient they cannot be treated unless they pay for it out of pocket. As Jay points out,

> Right, so most patients have no idea about the details of their coverage or what's in their insurance plan. When they meet their limit of the number of treatments or if they have to pay out of pocket for copays or whatever, I get to be the one that tells them. So I'm the bad guy that has to say, "Hey, your insurance doesn't cover this and if you want me to treat you, you're going to have to give me the

> cash." It makes me look like I'm holding patients hostage, when it's really the insurance company putting the screws to them. But then I have to be the one that says, "Would you like to go to a cash system, where you pay me every time you come to the office?" It makes me feel like I'm a used car salesman even though I have every right to seek payment for my services. But patients start to look at me as if I'm pulling a fast one on them or I'm trying to take advantage of them in some way.

In reality, many patients are experiencing the impact of greater out-of-pocket expenses for treatment, whether it is at the chiropractor's office, the dentist's office, or with their primary care physician. Many Americans are beginning to realize the insurance they purchase does not cover much of their needs on a regular basis. What makes it a bit different with a chiropractor is that there can be an underlying question or even a suspicion about the motives of the chiropractor. It is almost as if they wonder if they are being exploited. As, Theresa, a chiropractic patient, stated,

> I don't know why, but when the chiropractor I used to visit told me this, I wondered if he was telling me the truth. I don't really know the details of my insurance plan, I don't think most people do. But I didn't have a problem when my dentist told me my insurance didn't cover a LOT of the costs of my crown. And I didn't really think much about paying a lot out-of-pocket for my MRI last year. But for some reason, I had that little pause of disbelief when my chiropractor told me that my plan only covered a certain number of visits and I had to pay for everything after that. Is that wrong? Is it because chiropractors have a reputation for being a little shifty and maybe a little desperate? I don't know, but I remember starting to question a lot more about what my chiropractor charged me for after that.

It was not uncommon during the study to encounter patients who offered similar observations as Theresa in describing their particular provider. Perhaps there is an underlying suspicion or question about the motives of chiropractors, even if it is unfounded. The realities, though, are that this can translate into a loss of business for the chiropractors—either from the loss of patients if the mistrust is serious, or simply the challenges of running and sustaining a practice in light of the reduced reimbursement rates and limits on visits by insurance companies. More than a few chiropractors in the study mentioned the inevitability of going to a cash model, but most are very afraid to do so. As Doug points out,

> Man, it would sure make things easier for me, but I don't think I could do it and not lose too many patients. They just want to use their insurance, and I don't blame them . . . that's what they pay premiums for—but I would love to go to

a cash model and not have to deal with insurance companies—I just don't think I can do it and I know a lot of my friends who are chiropractors feel the same way. It's scary.

The cash model is something that is not as popular in traditional medicine—most physicians, who are experiencing the same challenges from insurance companies with regard to reimbursement rates and administrative challenges, are also quite reluctant to opt for a cash only model. At the same time, however, most of the practice-building seminars that target chiropractors embrace the idea of a cash only system. Also, as was mentioned in a previous chapter, franchises like the Joint operate exclusively on a cash system. So there is some reason to consider this as a strategy, particularly since most chiropractors and physicians do not believe that reimbursement rates are going to increase in the future.

The challenges relating to low reimbursement rates, the administrative issues to managing the front office as well as treating patients, along with the other administrative tasks in running a practice, increase the chances that a provider will make a mistake with billing or, worse, the desperation felt by declining revenue leads them to take shortcuts or gamble that they will not get caught in billing insurance companies for fees. This tendency inevitably leads to a discussion of Medicare and insurance fraud.

MEDICARE FRAUD, AUDITS, AND ACCOUNTABILITY

I am sitting in a chiropractor's office waiting for patients to be treated when Joe comes into the waiting room in a panic. He says, "I need to show you something, come on into my office." We walk back to a small room just off of the receptionist's area and he shows me a notice from the Medicare office, asking for information about patients. He says the following:

> This is what I am dealing with now. I had a patient complain about paying for treatments he received like six months ago. I haven't seen the guy since then but he filed a complaint. Now Medicare wants to see my clinical notes for him and five other patients. I have heard about these audits and it scares the crap out of me! They can do anything they want and the fines are like $10,000 or more! I found this [hands me another printout] online from a colleague. He's a chiropractor who advises people like me how to handle an inquiry or an audit. I haven't slept in three days because of this—not only is it a pain in the rear to get all that information together, I am worried that they'll find some little thing wrong and then they'll want more information on more patients. I have heard this becomes a never-ending series of requests from them. . . . And you can't really complain. I just don't know what I'm going to do. I treated this guy

> for his work-related injury and then he stopped coming. So I know I didn't do anything wrong.

During this conversation, Joe's wife, who works in the practice with him, along with one other staff person, offers her opinions about Medicare. She says the following:

> Of all the groups to go after with audits, they go after the little guys. The chiropractors. Why? Because they know we can't really fight them and they can do whatever they want to us. I don't see them going after doctors like they go after chiropractors. It's typical of how we are treated.

This issue of Medicare audits and its accountability measures are one of several issues in health care reform that has impacted chiropractors. At the time of Joe's wife's comments, I had just finished reading a report issued by the Office of Inspector General, a division of the Department of Health and Human Services, the overseeing agency for health programs like Medicare and Medicaid. In that report, it cited that of all the providers who were cited for fraud, abuse, and errors in Medicare billing, chiropractors were overwhelmingly the largest set of offenders. In fact, the report showed that for 2013, an estimated $359 million in Medicare payments for chiropractic services did not comply with Medicare requirements (Office of Inspector General, 2016).

The OIG Report

To begin, Medicare Part B covers chiropractic services for patients. Medicare requires that the services be provided by a qualified chiropractor and that they are reasonable and necessary for a patient's illness or injury. Medicare limits coverage to manual manipulation of the spine to correct a spinal subluxation, but it does not cover maintenance therapy.

To receive payment from Medicare, a chiropractor must document the services provided during the initial and subsequent visits as required by the Benefit Manual and the Local Coverage Determinations (LCD) for chiropractic services. Specifically, a chiropractor must specify the exact level of subluxation. Depending on the five regions of the spine (cervical, thoracic, lumbar, sacrum, or coccyx), the chiropractor may bill Medicare for treatment using one of three Current Procedural Terminology (CPT) codes: 98940 (treatment of one or two regions; 98941 (treatment of three or four regions); and 98942 (treatment of all five regions of the spine).

The CMS provides that certain conditions may require as many as three months of treatment and that chronic conditions may need a longer time span for treatment. However, when no further improvement is seen or can be reasonably expected from continuous care, the treatment is considered maintenance therapy. To identify a patient's illness or injury as acute care, CMS requires that chiropractors note the abbreviation (AT—acute treatment) on a claim when providing corrective treatment for a subluxation. Without this designation or modifier, CMS will deny the claims on the basis that they are maintenance therapy. However, simply including the modifier does not automatically mean the service provided was needed. Chiropractors must document the justification for the services provided according to guidelines set out by CMS (Office of Inspector General, 2016).

The OIG selected a stratified sample of 105 chiropractic services based on the services offered and the date of those services during the 2013 calendar year. In their analysis of these services, the OIG found that most Medicare payments did not comply with the program's requirements. Of the 105 services sampled, only 11 were in compliance with Medicare requirements. In most cases, the documentation provided by the chiropractors did not support the medical necessity of the services and most were beyond the three-month time limit for services, which qualified as maintenance therapy. As it is defined by the Benefit Manual, maintenance therapy

> is a treatment plan that seeks to prevent disease, promote health, and prolong and enhance the quality of life or (2) therapy that is performed to maintain or prevent deterioration of a chronic condition? Acute subluxation (e.g. strains or sprains) problems may require as many as three months of treatment but some require very little treatment. . . . Chronic spinal joint condition[s] . . . may require a longer treatment time, but not with higher frequency." (Office of Inspector General, 2017:7)

The breakdown of the ninety-four chiropractic services that were not in compliance includes subluxation of the spine that were not present, was not treated, or both; manual manipulation of the spinal subluxation was maintenance therapy or was not appropriate for treatment of the patient's condition or both; and manual manipulation of the spinal subluxation would not be expected to result in improvement within a reasonable and generally predictable period of time.

Extrapolating from the sample results, the OIG estimates that approximately $358.8 million or about 82 percent of the $438 million paid by Medicare for chiropractic services was inappropriately paid to chiropractors. The report states that clearly the AT modifier and the listing of the initial treatment dates did not prevent chiropractors from performing medically unnecessary chiropractic services to patients. Instead, chiropractors routinely assigned the AT modifier to virtually all of their patients, whether the treatment was for treatment of a subluxation or not. The report states that all but twenty-nine of the seventeen million chiropractic services included in their review contained the AT modifier.

Additionally, while documentation was provided by chiropractors in the respective patient files, they did not document the medical necessity of the services as outlined in the guidelines by Medicare. The OIG report also noted that despite a great deal of effort to inform chiropractors of these requirements and how to properly submit claims for medically necessary treatment, many chiropractors billed for services that did not meet Medicare requirements. The report concludes that CMS could have saved Medicare more than $358 million if it had effective controls that resulted in payment for medically necessary chiropractic services. The high error rate (82 percent) indicates that chiropractors are billing inappropriately, whether intentionally with the hope of not getting caught, a belief that what they are treating is not maintenance therapy, or because they simply do not understand the coding and billing process.

This is not the first time that the OIG has discovered improprieties with the payment for chiropractic services. OIG conduced four separate reviews, with reports issued between 2013 and 2016, and have consistently found that either payments for chiropractic services were medically unnecessary, incorrectly coded, insufficiently documented, or not documented at all, resulting in overpayments in the millions of dollars. In 2005, for instance, the OIG issued a report that stated:

> As chiropractic care extends beyond 12 treatments in a year, it becomes increasingly likely that individual services are medically unnecessary. The likelihood of a service being medically unnecessary increases even more significantly after 24 treatments. (Office of Inspector General, 2013: 9)

In 2013, the OIG analyzed claims totaling $502 million for chiropractic services and found that Medicare paid $76 million for questionable claims and nearly $21 million for claims that did not meet Medicare requirements. Each time OIG made recommendations to CMS regarding a more reliable system of control and accountability to address the problem of maintenance therapy by chiropractors. CMS attempted to implement a prior authorization medical review of services by certain chiropractors. OIG disagreed with this conclusion, citing that only a small group of chiropractors who were repeat offenders would be identified for dubious billing practices or claims that were denied, but these offenders might not be the ones who are receiving payment for maintenance therapy.

Thus, while it is understandable that Joe's wife might feel a bit persecuted, as do many chiropractors about their scope of practice, their philosophy, and their inability to succeed in practice, it is unclear whether or not the federal government is singling out chiropractors for audits. Instead, it might be the case, and some of the documentation supports such a position, that the federal government has a duty and obligation to address issues they are aware of in the distribution of taxpayer dollars. Jenny, a chiropractor involved in the study, noted the following:

> They (chiropractors) know what they are doing. They are just hoping they don't get flagged. These are not stupid people who can't figure out that they only get a limited number of treatments per patient. What they are trying to do is get as many treatments as they can before they get caught. Medicare has given them lots of information and shown them again and again that they can't bill for maintenance therapy. But these guys just keep doing it anyway. It's part of what's wrong with medicine in this country, so much money is spent on waste and improper payments to doctors.
>
> Chiropractors are getting a lot of attention because there are only so many things they can code for—whereas a primary care physician has a lot more codes to choose from so it's a lot harder to spot those irregularities. But everyone is doing it. And since chiropractors feel they have to make as much off every patient that walks in the door, they end up fudging the books by saying the treatments are for a new injury; that they're not doing maintenance therapy. That's a fine line because I can see what they are saying—if a guy gets treated for a back problem and then reinjures himself, that shouldn't count against the number of treatments for the first injury.
>
> But then again, ten or twelve visits is a lot of treatment time. I will get crucified by my colleagues for saying that, but honestly? That's a lot. I should be able to get you up and running in one or two treatments if it's an injury. So even with another injury or the same one flaring up again, I should be able to stay within a twelve visit limit, or I should be able to document what's happening and justify it that way. But like so many things in this profession, too many guys push the limits and then they make it hard for everyone because now Medicare is suspicious of anybody doing chiropractic treatment, forgetting for the moment that preventative care is cheaper in the long run for the government—but those are the rules of the game and we should be playing by them. But many of us are not, sad to say.

If chiropractors, whether through intentional misrepresentation, outright fraudulent practices, or a lack of understanding of the coding and reimbursement procedures, are disproportionately represented in the improper submission of fees for services, an investigation and greater scrutiny is absolutely the most appropriate course of action. That said, what remains unclear are the steps involved in that auditing process and if the rules are evenly applied in all cases.

Determining Mistakes and Fraud

Consistent with the idea that there needs to be greater accountability in medicine, the CMS have added programs and contractors to examine providers' claims and identify errors and overpayments. CMS contracted with what area known as Recovery Audit Contractors (RACs) to identify Medicare overpayments and underpayments and to have those providers return fees to Medicare. RACs review claims submitted by medical providers and attempt to identify instances where they were either overpaid for services or underpaid for them. RACs are paid on a contingency basis, meaning they are paid based on how many claims they identify as inappropriate. The RAC program also now includes Medicaid claims and other dimensions of Medicare, including Medicare Advantage (Part C) and Prescription Drug plans (Part D) (Wachler and Associates, 2017).

CMS has also created Medicare Administrative Contractors (MACs) who handle enrollment issues and claims processing. They are also responsible for addressing billing errors and incorrectly coded bills. MACs also review claims to determine if proper amounts were paid to providers and adjust or even deny payments that they deem unreasonable or not medically necessary for patients. For those providers who have excessively high error rates or those who have consistently been overpaid, they are put on a payment plan to reimburse Medicare. One tool used by MACs is the Comprehensive Error Rate Testing Program (CERT).

This program is designed to determine the reasons for claim errors and to develop a concrete plan to improve compliance by providers. The CERT contractor randomly selects a sample of Medicare claims and requests medical records and documentation from the provider who submitted those claims. While the goal is to understand the reasons for the errors in the first place, once the provider submits the information to CERT, if an overpayment or underpayment is discovered, CERT sends this information to the MAC for recovery (Wachler and Associates, 2017).

Given that there is a line between mistakes and outright fraud, CMS has also created Zone Program Integrity Contractors (ZPICs), who are responsible for identifying suspected fraud. This program is different from MACs, which are designed to identify and correct errors in billing. ZPICs use a variety of proactive techniques, including computer-generated algorithms to identify providers who exceed an estimated rate of claims for a given code in a particular geographic region. This benchmark is then used to identify providers who exceed these expectations. ZPICs then issues a request for additional information about bills submitted for reimbursement. This can be a time-consuming process and often requires detailed information from the provider, which is then reviewed for accuracy and approval of the claim.

In addition to their own analysis, ZPICs often receive referrals from MACS and RACs about particular claims (Wachler and Associates, 2017).

In those instances where a contractor has determined an error or overpayment, and if a particular provider does not agree with the finding of the RAC, the MAC or the ZPIC, they may file an appeal.

Chiropractors' Experiences with Audits

Mike experienced an audit for the first time during the study. He says the following:

> Hey, I'm up at night about this. I have been told this is no joke and the fines are like $10,000, even if you didn't do anything wrong. There are law firms out there that specialize in protecting chiropractors and doctors from these types of audits, but they're expensive too. So either way it costs you a lot of money. I did my best to give them all the records and notes that I had, but sometimes they go after you for not having a signature on the form, or some other minor thing. That's not what this should be about. You should be going after the guys that are bilking the system and trying to defraud the taxpayer out of money for not treating patients or padding the bill with things you didn't do. Not hitting the little guy hard for forgetting a signature or inadvertently putting in the wrong code. I'm going to give them everything they asked for, but I will tell you, this creates a lot of stress for me—I can't afford to take a hit like that or to pay back reimbursements on patients when I legitimately treated them. That money is already spent on the practice. As it is, I'm already on the margins so I can't afford any major expense like this or worse, be put on some list that flags me for more attention than other guys.

Dave talks about his experiences with an audit. He says part of the challenge involves Medicare not understanding that patients often come to see him for different injuries. He says the following:

> But the same thing with Medicare . . . you get the letter every quarter that tells you the average patient visit is here and you've seen this patient x amount of time . . . and I'm like, "yeah, I saw them in January and February for a neck problem and now I'm seeing him for a back problem." Even though it is supposed to be visits per condition, they combine it to per patient per year, so it skews everything to make it look like I'm exceeding the number of visits allowed. [What does that do? Is it a problem because you're then more likely to get audited and they ask you for patient information and documentation of what you did?]
>
> I've been audited two times by Medicare. And the first time it was because for our adjustment codes, we have five regions of the body. And you bill based on one to two regions, three to four regions or five regions. Right? So what they

did in each region of the state, they took, the top 20 percent for each of these categories and asked to see their records. So I was selected because I have quite a few Medicare patients. So I sent it in and they sent it back and I think my grade at that time was like a 74% or something like that. So I got that and called them up and asked the lady, "So how did I end up with this percentage?" And she told me "Part of it was because you didn't have the specific level of what you adjusted." And I'm like, "It's right there in my notes, it's very specific. It's right there."

And she said, "Oh yeah, you're right. And that's a major thing right there." So I said, "Does that change the grade?" And she says, "Well it's too late." I'm like "What do you mean it's too late?" And she's like, "Well it's already in the system." And then she says, "Listen, you got one of the highest scores. A lot of you guys are . . . most of the scores, and it should be an embarrassment for you guys, because most of the scores are in the 20–30 percent."

They're just not paying attention, they're just checking things off, which defeats the purpose. But the kicker was that after talking to her about it, she said "Just make these changes and you'll be fine." And she was in her 60s and a retired nurse, she said "Because you didn't get above an 80% you're probably going to get audited again." And I'm like, "But I did it the right way!" And sure enough, two years later, I get audited again.

So about two years after that, I get audited again. I paid back Medicare like $250 or something and it wasn't a large one, like twelve or twenty patients over a twelve-month period of time . . . out of those ones they took? That got denied, it was in a short period of time. . . . And it was I had some that got denied on the second visit, some I had 21 or 22 times, but they were way down the ten allowable. . . . But the system kicked it out. So for me, it's like, as soon as you kicked that one out shouldn't all of those that followed get kicked out too? But no, it's just those on those dates. The visits before and the visits after were paid. So I asked the guy. And he said "If you're appealing this" . . . and I was like, "No, no, no, I'm not appealing. I just want some clarification on this, because the last time this happened, I talked to the lady and she gave me some guidance." And the guy goes, "Well, just do everything the lady told you" . . . and I'm like, "I did!"

Cisco points out that the problem is not really about billing, it is much more fundamental to the scope of practice for chiropractors. He says the following:

I think it is completely inappropriate for an insurance company to determine what's in the patient's best interest. I believe in the idea of maintenance therapy because I've seen it work. But when insurance companies, who have never been to chiropractic college, start telling me that they won't pay because they don't believe in the idea of maintenance therapy, I have to call them out on that. Who is the expert here? I've been audited several times and while I would like to be honest and describe exactly what I'm doing, I know that if I use the term maintenance therapy I'm not going to get paid. So do I game

> the system? Absolutely, and I don't think there is anything wrong with that. Are you going to tell me that doctors don't fudge the forms to fit the little box they need to get paid? Of course they do. But the problem isn't really about whether I'm gaming the system or not. The problem is that the insurance companies think they can practice medicine because they hold the purse strings and we don't. So if I am doing what I think it right for my patients but have to manipulate the process to do that, then I don't lose sleep at night over it. If I get caught, I get caught, but what I think you found is that most chiropractors feel like I do.

Jake is less than tolerant of the process, citing the fact that Medicare continues to change the rules. He says the following:

> I can't seem to figure out what I'm doing wrong. Just when I get a clear answer from people about what it is I am supposed to be doing, I get notified that I have done something wrong. How can the rules change so quickly without notice and yet I'm getting hammered because I thought I was doing it properly?

Mike takes a different approach to the billing problem. He says the following:

> Hey, the system doesn't work and everyone involved in it knows that. I'm hoping that by creating a problem, someone pays attention to how fundamentally unfair it is towards chiropractors. I know chiropractors may be engaging in fraud, but in some ways the money justifies the amount of time they have to spend collecting all the crazy information they require to get reimbursed.

Tanya expresses concerns about the lack of effective accountability. She says the following:

> No one is paying close attention to what happens. Even with all the controls in place, a lot of chiropractors feel like everyone has been asleep at the switch, so they just keep billing as they always have and hope they don't get caught. The secret to all of this is to know what data they are using and to fly under the wire. If you overbill or you always bill at the highest rate, you're going to get caught. But for the most part, no one really pays attention to what you submit if you say the right things on the charts and you don't try to take advantage of how the system works.

It seems clear from some of the comments of providers that there exists a good bit of confusion about what is expected of chiropractors in terms of meeting or exceeding the limits of Medicare requirements regarding adjustments. There also seems to be some misunderstanding of how cases are selected and the questions asked of providers. For many, they do not see that the sample selected, like any sample, does not take into account all of the possible cases or patients seen in a given month, which would explain why some treatments are paid and others are questioned.

It may be that the way it was explained to chiropractors has led many to believe that there would be a consistency to the process, where any cases over a certain number would be identified and queries would be made. However, since the system identifies cases in a certain window and only a certain number, those cases and only those cases are flagged. But there could be others that the system does not identify that are similar in nature to the ones that are questioned.

There is also an element of the human factor at work as well. As this last account illustrated, even when mistakes are made, it could be that the contract employees may not be able to access the system to change the error. It may also be the case that some employees may not wish to call attention to the mistake and simply move forward, even though the provider did everything that was asked of him. These types of problems only exacerbate the tension between providers and insurance companies and could easily lead to providers attempting to remedy an injustice by engaging in further misbehavior.

DISCUSSION

In his classic text, entitled *The Sociological Imagination*, sociologist C. Wright Mills (1959) offers an important distinction between personal troubles and public issues. The former refers to a social problem in society, such as poverty, that impacts a person based on their individual decisions. Thus, the reason why people are poor is a result of their inability to create or maintain a strong work ethic, a lack of talent, drive, motivation, or some other characteristic of that individual or group of individuals, that keeps them from being successful. Thus, the explanation of the problem resides in the individuals affected by it.

In contrast, public issues explain a social problem as a result of elements embedded in the social structure, culture or organization of society. To use the previous example, people are poor not because they are lazy or unwilling to do what is necessary to succeed, but because of structural barriers, such as inadequate educational systems in some neighborhoods, a labor market that only provides low-paying jobs that do not carry health benefits, or racial discrimination, that keep some groups of people from succeeding.

Mills felt that many problems are often understood as personal troubles or individual challenges, but in reality, structural factors often play a greater role in understanding the problems' scope and complexity. This appreciation for the structural basis to what appear to be individual challenges Mills termed *the sociological imagination.* In describing how to understand and use the sociological imagination, Mills says, when a large group of people are impacted, it is unreasonable to think only in terms of individual talent, motivation, or discipline to explain the problem. He says the following: "The very structure of opportunities has collapsed. Both the correct statement of the problem and the range of possible solutions require us to consider the economic and political institutions of the society, and not merely the personal situation and character of a scatter of individuals" (p. 9).

Mills (1959) offers valuable insight into understanding how social policy impacts and is impacted by the causes of social problems. One could even extend this line of thinking a bit further and assign political views based on the dichotomy that Mills offers, with liberals tending to explain social problems on the basis of structural explanations (public issues), whereas more conservative approaches tend to explain social problems at a more individual level (personal troubles).

Mills's (1959) ideas about personal troubles versus public issues can easily be applied to the discussion of the health care debate going on in the United States. At the heart of the debate over health care reform is the larger question of whether health care is considered a right or a privilege in this country. As some experts have noted, if one views health care as a privilege, it is also consistent with the idea that people are responsible for themselves and their family. Arguing from a paradigm sometimes referred to as *personal attribution*, the idea here is that the reason people are poor or disadvantaged is because they lack the talent or drive to succeed or have a sense of entitlement that prevents them from making the important decisions that contribute to their success. Health care is simply another example of this perspective and if people want medical treatment, they should pay for it. This argument does not assert that the poor are undeserving of medical care, rather it contends that the best way to help the poor is to provide them with jobs so that they can purchase the health insurance they need, just like everyone else. But providing high quality health care without addressing the larger issues that stem from poverty means that the poor are likely to always need help from the government. Thus, in the same way that people make decisions about how to spend their money, some will choose to spend it on something besides quality health care.

The other side of this debate, sometimes referred to as *systemic attribution*, suggesting that elements built into the system itself, are responsible for some of the problems the poor and others experience. That is, while people do make choices about the importance of eating right, exercising, and taking preventive steps to remain healthy, some health problems are beyond an individual's control. Genetics plays a role in a person's health, their exposure to disease, the environment they live in, as well as the information they receive about health concerns. For instance, the use of tobacco and the health effects of cigarette smoking were not known to the public for decades, largely because the tobacco industry kept that information concealed and generally misled the public about its deleterious effects. Thus, while it may be reasonable to suggest that individuals bear the responsibility for their own health based on individual choices, people are not always fully informed of the risks or consequences of their lifestyle choices and some health problems are not controllable with attention to things like eating right and exercising.

This argument of health care as a right is said by some observers to be a fundamental way for society to define its core values. Some experts note that society has an ethical obligation to create and deliver equitable access to treatment by making care a right. Given health care's special place in society, as evidenced by the fact that the right to health care is recognized by all Western countries except the United States, ensures that every citizen should have some type of national health insurance. In contrast, the United States has a large segment of the population who are significantly impacted in a negative way as health care costs rise, more than what the average person can afford. Under the current model, it also appears that purchasing insurance for these needs is beyond the reach of many Americans.

In another sense, the idea of health care as a right stands in stark contrast to the idea of a capitalist society, which, by definition, contains elements of inequality. However, as some experts point out, the creation of a welfare state, one that is characterized by its guarantees to its citizens (e.g., the freedom of expression, freedom of the press, of religion, of assembly, equality before the law, to vote, to protest, etc.) emerged at about the same time as the rise of modern capitalism. In the modern welfare state, it is not the ownership and control of private property, but the rights of citizenship that assures the rights of its people.

Given the enormous success that the United States has experienced as a result of embracing capitalist principles, some people, particularly those who can afford to pay for health care, may feel that such a shift is incompatible with democracy and with the things that made this country great. Thus, the health care reform discussion may be less about the spiraling costs of health care and more about something much more fundamental and central to what it means to be a citizen in the United States.

However, the idea of health care as a right instead of a privilege is based on the ideas of fundamental fairness and concern for basic rights for all members of American society. The fact that other countries that espouse such a view, and themselves advocates of capitalism and freedoms, makes the argument for a similar model in the United States a compelling one.

While many chiropractors in this study lament about the challenges that health care reform in general, and Obamacare in particular, are having on their ability to sustain their practices, they are not the only ones impacted by the changes to medicine and managed care. In fact, in a 2014 article in the journal *Medical Economics*, citing the top fifteen challenges facing all physicians, many of the issues identified include compliance with showing improved patient outcomes as a result of treatment, declining reimbursements for care under the Affordable Care Act, an increased level of dissatisfaction with the profession and burnout, along with the rising costs of maintaining a practice and other issues relating to managed care (Terry et al., 2014).

Increasingly, physicians are finding the idea of simply working for a hospital more attractive than the independence and autonomy of having their own private practice. With regard to job satisfaction, many physicians are feeling the effects of being pushed out of practicing medicine and simply catering to insurance companies and patients, who see them merely as prescription writers who will give patients the medications they want to solve their immediate problems. As Jake pointed out in one discussion, he thinks chiropractors and physicians have a lot in common when it comes to satisfaction levels. He says the following:

> Why do you think so many doctors will say they don't recommend being a doctor to their kids? Can't make any money and they're not enjoying, they're not seeing the results. So let's say, you come to me and say "I have this issue, I think I have a sinus infection." But I think it's a bacterial problem. "Here's your script." And then you never come back. So the job satisfaction isn't there and you truly don't know if what you did worked.

Thus, in many ways, the challenges of health care reform are impacting chiropractors and physicians in similar ways. Whether it is a physician in family practice or a chiropractor working on his or her own, the viability of solo practitioners is questionable in an industry that is moving toward the merging of smaller practices and greater specialization. This latter trend, as we have seen, has some advantages, but one has to question whether it really benefits most patients with the more common types of illnesses and injuries. Either way, specialization creates a gap in the primary care provider market.

One solution that has been proposed, is to elevate the status and training of physician assistants and nurse practitioners, who can then take on some of the initial diagnoses for routine matters that are now being handled by primary care physicians. Given that they already have substantial training, such an expansion of their role may be a viable option in the future. In many states nurse practitioners already have prescription drug rights and many physician assistants have been prescribing drugs to patients for years. What appears less likely, despite the efforts of many chiropractic colleges and Reformists, is that chiropractors will become the next iteration of primary care providers. The public does not currently see them as general practitioners, their training does not adequately prepare them to fill that role, and it is unlikely that the medical community would support such a transition given the current state of affairs in the chiropractic profession.

As was mentioned, chiropractors are, in the vast majority of cases, solo practitioners. This fact, coupled with the changes in health care in general, with managed care resulting in a greater use of physicians as hospital employees, there remain real questions about the place for chiropractors in medicine. This is true regardless of where one stands on the debate about the effectiveness of chiropractic care. It also seems clear that the future of medicine requires the public to pay for more of their health care needs out of pocket, and given the stagnation in incomes for most Americans, the funds that may be currently dedicated to chiropractic care will compete with other medical needs, even if people understand that they need to take better care of themselves. At some point, they are going to need to see a physician for something and may not have the money to spend on both forms of treatments. This is true despite the commonality of back and neck pain—patients are going to need a wide range of care and chiropractors have not made a convincing argument that they can holistically treat patients for all things. This is particularly true with those chiropractors that argue maintenance care is needed to remain healthy.

As we have seen, some patients pause when their chiropractor tells them they need to be seen regularly in order to remain healthy. This is not the case with other medical providers, or if they do, the treatments are not as frequent with dentists or other providers. This perception is also reinforced since the idea of maintenance therapy has not been proven to be effective or needed—even many chiropractors contend that this is based more on financial incentives than medical necessity. As health care costs continue to rise and resources remain a challenge for most Americans, chiropractic care may be something that people curtail when more pressing expenses occur. As out-of-pocket expenses for routine medical care increase, this may happen sooner than later, particularly as insurance plans require higher premiums, deductibles and copays. Such a mixture of events will likely have a catastrophic effect on the chiropractic profession. Unlike physicians, however, chiropractors generally do not have the option of becoming an employee of a hospital or other entity. This may be one of the reasons why chiropractic colleges have attempted to identify a need in the market, the shortage of primary care physicians, and attempt to fill it by redefining the profession to be more like first-line providers. This may work, but as was mentioned, medicine already has two types of mid-level providers who can step into that gap: physician assistants and nurse practitioners. The added attraction to using members of these professions is that they are already considered mainstream medical providers and have a wide range of skill sets that run parallel to what physicians already do. They would need some additional training, of course, but they seem better poised to fill the shortage than chiropractors, who tend to be seen more as specialists. Thus there remain some real questions about the role of chiropractors in the future of medicine.

What is fairly clear is that the current model used by most chiropractors is simply unsustainable, as health care and the insurance industry have changed the trajectory of medicine, along with the public's need for convenience and simplicity to meet their health needs. Solutions such as a cash system, seem more like stop-gap measures to the insurance challenge than a larger discussion of what role, if any, should and could chiropractic play. This is particularly true in light of the aging of America.

NOTE

1. At the same time, half of the population has little or no health care costs, which accounts for about 3 percent of the spending.

REFERENCES

Adams, S. "Why Do So Many Doctors Regret Their Job Choice?" *Forbes*, April 27th. Available at https://www.forbes.com/sites/susadams/2012/04/27/why-do-so-many-doctors-regret- their-job-choice/#10521d8c371fa

Alonzo-Zaldivar, R. 2016. "$10,345 per person: U.S. health care spending reaches new peak." *Associated Press*, July 13th, available at http://www.pbs.com/newshour/rundown/new-peak-us-health-care-spending-10345-per-person/

Bagley, N. 2017. "Trump's Ominous Threat to Withhold Payment From Health Insurers, Explained." *Vox,* April 27th. Available at https://www.vox.com/the-big-idea/2017/3/29/15107836/lawsuit-aca-payments-reimbursement-unconstitutional

Bloomberg, 2017. "Donald Trump Hints at Ending Subsidy that Gives Health Care to the Poor." *Fortune*, July 29th. Available at http://fortune.com/2017/07/29/Donald-trump-affordable-care-act-subsidy

Brinkley, D. 1998. *Out of Retirement*. New York: Vintage.

Bryan, B. 2017a. "Three States Proved That One Move From Trump Could Send Healthcare Costs Skyrocketing for Millions of Americans." *Business Insider,* August 1st. Available at http://www.msn.com/en-us/news/us/3-states-proved-that-one-move-from-trump-could-send-healthcare-costs-skyrocketing-for-millions-of-americans/arAApgu74?li=BBmkt5R&ocid=spartandhp

Bryan, B. 2017. "It Just Became Harder for Trump to Blow Up Obamacare." *Yahoo News*, August 2nd. Available at http://www.yahoo.com/finance/news/just-became-harder-trump- blwo-140735935.html

"CBO: 20% Premium Rise Without Obamacare Insurance Subsidies." *Newsline*. August 15th. Available at https://newsline.com/cbo-20-premium-rise-without-obamacare-insurance-subsidies

Cox, C., Claxton, G., and Levitt, L. 2015. "Analysis of Insurer Participation in 2016 Marketplaces." *Kaiser Family Foundation*, November 3rd. Available at http://www.kff.org/health-reform/issue-brief/analysis-of-insurer-participation-in-2016-marketplaces

Davis, E. 2017. "DRG 101: What is it and how does it work?" *Verywell*, August 13th. Available at https://www.verywell.com/drg-101-what-is-a-drg-how-does-it-work-3916755.

Fromson, J. A. 2011. "Physician Shortages in the Specialties Taking a Toll." *Journal of the New England Journal of Medicine Network*, October 31st. Available at http://www.nejmcareercenter.org/article/physician-shortages-in-the-specialities-taking-a-toll

Hamblin, J. 2015. "What Doctors Make" *The Atlantic,* January 27. Available at https://www.theatlantic.com/health/archive/2015/01/physician-salaries/384846

Kessler, G. 2017. "President Trump's Claim of Obamacare 'bailouts' for Insurance Companies." *Washington Post*, August 7th. Available at https://www.washingtonpost.com/news/fact-checker/wp/2017/08/07/president-trumps-claim-of-obamacare-bailouts-for-insurance-companies/?utm_term=.3b29daab5ce7

Laszewski, R. 2016. "Trump Wants to Keep the Obamacare Pre-Existing Conditions Reforms—He First Said So in February." *Forbes*, November 12. Available at https://www.forbes.com/sites/robertlaszewski2/2016/11/12/isnt-news-that-trump-wants-to-keep-the-pre-existin-condition-reforms-he-said-so-in-february/#6e9eb2621d48

Liptak, J. 2012. "Supreme Court Upholds Health Care Law 5-4 in Victory for Obama." *New York Times*, June 28. Available at http://www.nytimes.com/2012/6/29/US/Supreme-Court-lets-healthcare-law-largely-stand.html

Mills, C. W. 1959. *The Sociological Imagination*. New York: Oxford University Press.

Moffitt, R. 1993. *A Guide to the Clinton Health Plan*. Washington, DC: The Heritage Foundation. Available at http://www.heritage.org/health-care-reform/report/guide-the-clinton-health-plan

National Conference of State Legislatures. 2017. *Affordable Care Act Medicaid Expansion.* Available at http://www.ncsi.org/research/health/affordable-care-act-expansion.aspx

Nichols, J. 2017. "Single Payer is a Rational Health Care System." *The Nation*, September 13. Available at https://www.thenation.com/article/single-payer-is-a-rational-health-care-system-an-exclusive-interview-with-bernie-sanders-on-his-medicare-for-all-plan/

O'Donnell, J., Hoyer, M., and Alcindor, Y. 2014. "Some Chiropractors Making Big Medicare-paid Adjustments." *USA Today*, April 29. Available at https://www.usatoday.com/story/news/politics/2014/04/29/medicare-data-chiropractors-reimbursements/7720741

Parks, M., Rogin, A. Parkinson, J. and Caplan, D. 2017. "Skinny Obamacare Repeal Fails in Senate Vote." *ABC News*. July 28. Available at http://www.abcnews.com/politics/gop-skinny-repeal-option-health-care/story?id=48870581

Peterson Foundation, 2017. Infographic: U.S. Healthcare Spending. Available at http://www.pgpf.org/infographic/infographic-us-healthcare-spending

Punke, H. 2013. "Survey: 42% of Physicians are Dissatisfied." *Jackson Healthcare*. Available at http://www.beckershospitalreview.com/hospital-physician-relationships/survey-42-of-physicians-are-dissatisfied.html

Rabin, R. C. 2014. "Burnt Out Primary Care Docs Are Voting with their Feet." *Kaiser Health News*, April 1st. Available at http://www.Khn.org/news/doctor-burnout

"Republicans Question Legality of Obamacare Payments to Insurance Companies." *Washington Free Beacon*, June 11th, 2014, available at http://freebeacon.com/issues/-question-legality-of-obamacare-payments-to-insurance-companies

Riley, R. 2017. Bill Clinton: Domestic Affairs. Charlottesville, VA: University of Virginia Miller Center. Available at https://millercenter.org/president/clinton/domestic-affairs

Schumock, G. T., Li, E. C., Wiest, M. D., Suda, K. J., Stubbings, J., Matusiak, L., Hunkler, R., and Vemereuleun, L. C. 2017. "National Trends in Prescription Drug Expenditures and Projections for 2017." *American Journal of Health System Pharmacy* August, 74(15): 1158–1173. Available at https://doi.org/10.2146/ajhp170164

Schectman, J. 2017. "Trump Threatens to End Insurance Payments if No Healthcare Bill." *Reuters,* July 29th. Available at https://www.reuters.com/article/us-usa-healthcare-trump-idUSKBN1AE0QQ

Schencker, L. 2014. "Republicans file their suit against the Affordable Care Act." *Modern Healthcare*, November 21st. Available at http://www.modernhealthcare.com/article/20141121/NEWS/311219970

Spakovsky, H. 2015. "Several States Launch New Lawsuit Against Obamacare: Here's Why It Will Likely Go to the Supreme Court." *The Daily Signal,* October 21st. Available at http://www.dailysignal.com/2015/10/21/several-states-launch-new-lawsuit-against-obamacare-heres-why-it-will-go-to-the-supreme-court

Terry, K., Ritchie, A., Marbury, D., Smith, L., and Pofeldt, E. 2015. "Top 15 Challenges Facing Physicians in 2015." Medical Economics, December 1st. Available at http://www.medicaleconomics.com/editors-choice-me/top-15-challenges-facing-physicians-2015

The Henry J. Kaiser Family Foundation. 2015. The Facts on Medicare Spending and Financing. Available at http://www.kff.org/medicare/fact-sheet/medicare-spending-and-financing-fact-sheet

Updegrove, M. 2012. *Indomitable Will*. New York: Crown.

U.S. Department of Health and Human Services, Office of Inspector General, 2016. *Hundreds of Millions in Medicare Payments for Chiropractic Services Did Not Comply with Medicare Requirements*. Available at https://oig.hhs.gov/oas/reports/region9/91402033.pdf

Wachler and Associates. *Healthcare Audit Lawyers*. Available at https://www.wachler.com/healthcare-audit-lawyers.html

Waldman, D. 2014. "Single Payer is Root Cause of VA Deaths." *American Thinker*, June 4th. Available at http://www.americanthinker.com/articles/2014/06/single_payer_is_root_cause_of_va_deaths.html

"Who Will Win the Presidency?" 2016. *FiveThirtyEight*. Available at https://projects.fivethirtyeight.com/2016-election-forecast

Woodyard, C. and Layton, M. J. 2016. "Massive Price Increase on EpiPens Raise Alarm." *USA Today*, August 22nd. Available at https://www.usatoday.com/story/money/business/2016/08/22/two-senators-urge-scrutiny-epipen-price-boost/89129620/

Zernike, K. 2017. "The Hidden Subsidy that Helps Pay for Health Insurance." *New York Times,* July 7th. Available at https://www.nytimes.com/2017/07/07/health/health-insurance-tax-deduction.html

Chapter 8

Conclusion

As was mentioned in the opening chapter, the popularity of complementary and alternative medicine has increased in recent years (Report Linker, 2017). There may be many reasons for this, including dissatisfaction with the limits of traditional medicine, but sociologically, the pursuit of unconventional solutions to health problems can be framed by how people generally attempt to understand the world around them. As Festinger (1954) pointed out over sixty years ago, because there is a great deal of ambiguity in the social world, in that we do not always know what people are thinking or what motivates them to act a certain way, individuals attempt to find answers through indicators or cues, and when enough cues emerge, we are able to create a category that frames our understanding of people and their actions. Festinger points out that people have a fundamental "need to know" or understand the world around them.

The problem is that with the pace of life and the speed with which things change in the modern world, there is less time to delve deeply into an understanding of society and the people in it. As a result, in addition to creating broad typologies to classify people and events, we also draw conclusions or explanations of people and things. This classification and simple theories to explain life is part of what Heider (1958) referred to as a larger *naïve psychology* (Heider, 1958).

Such an understanding of how people process information and stimuli can be used to explain the growing popularity of alternative medicine. There remain a number of diseases, the causes of which remain unknown, and as we attempt to find ways to prevent illness, the answers are not always clear. The trust we place in physicians and others in health care remains a bit suspect, as has been the case since the 1800s, despite tremendous advances in medicine and technology. Thus, while we know more about medicine and illness than ever before, many people still get sick, even when they take all the necessary preventive steps. In the absence of a proven formula for health, and given the rising levels of dissatisfaction with traditional medicine, alternative medicine gives us some psychological relief that we are in control.

FRAMING CHIROPRACTIC MEDICINE SOCIOLOGICALLY

There are many issues related to chiropractic medicine, as the preceding chapters have noted and described in some detail. While it might be easy to simply conclude that the problems are intractable or that the personalities involved will limit the role of chiropractic medicine, chiropractors are neither the first nor the only profession that suffers from internal or external credibility problems.

One way to frame the discussion of the issues in chiropractic medicine is to draw from sociological theory. The work of Emile Durkheim and his explanation of the integration of society and its focus on social cohesion and trust help to explain what is happening with chiropractors and the profession.

Durkheim's Theory

At the most general and inclusive level, Durkheim's was a sociology of morality. At its most basic level, Durkheim's great concern was with the declining strength of the common morality in the modern world. People were in danger of what he called a "pathological loosening" of moral boundaries. These were important for without them, the individual would lose concern for others and simply pursue their passions (Coser, 1994).

We begin with a very complicated philosophical question: What is the basis for social order? If people are said to pursue rational self-interest, meaning they act in such a way that provides them with the things they need without regard for others, how is society possible? Why should people trust or cooperate with one another and not take advantage of each other should the circumstances permit? If one presumes that people are so selfish, then what holds society together?

Durkheim felt that the social order existed because of a common set of moral beliefs. This, he argued, allowed social contracts and economic relationships to form. Durkheim identified a special type of common moral beliefs as the *collective conscience*, and it is this framework that allows for a sense of trust to emerge. The collective conscience is a general belief or moral feeling that does not depend on any one person and creates a sense of trust that people will uphold their obligations and responsibilities to each other. The mutual trust that develops allows a solid and effective social order to emerge (Durkheim, 1997).

In his book, *The Division of Labor*, Durkheim describes what happened as a result of the Industrial Revolution, where much, if not all of society, was divided according to tenets of capitalism and the assembly line model of production. Gone were the simple agrarian societies, where people farmed the land. In its place were the city, the factory, and the massive influx of specific labor to produce products to be sold on the market for a profit. This not only had a significant impact on the economy, but on social life as well (Durkheim, 1997).

Durkheim based his analysis on two conceptualizations of society. The more primitive type, characterized by *Mechanical Solidarity*, has little or no division of labor. The more modern type, characterized by *Organic Solidarity*, has a much greater and more refined division of labor. People within primitive societies tend to occupy very general positions in which they perform a wide variety of tasks to handle a large number of responsibilities. In contrast, people who live in more modern societies occupy more specialized positions and have a much narrower range of tasks (Durkheim, 1997).

The changes in the division of labor have enormous implications for the structure of society and some of the more important implications are reflected in the differences between the two types of solidarity, and by extension, morality. A society characterized by mechanical solidarity is unified because everyone is essentially performing the same tasks. The bond among people is that they are all engaged in similar activities and have similar responsibilities. In contrast, a more modern society characterized by organic solidarity is held together by the fact that people have different tasks and responsibilities, but they need many others to survive (Durkheim, 1997).

Durkheim concluded that because individuals, groups, families, tribes, and so on perform virtually identical functions, they are likely to clash over these functions, especially if resources are scarce. The rise of the division of labor allows people and the social structures they create to complement, rather than conflict, with one another, and this in turn makes peaceful coexistence more likely. Furthermore, increasing the division of labor makes for greater efficiency with the result that resources increase and more and more people can survive peacefully. So while one might characterize the changes in society as problematic, Durkheim felt that there was a chance that good things could come from this shift in solidarity.

Durkheim attempted to pragmatically show this shift by examining the role and purpose of the law in society. Durkheim argued that in societies with mechanical solidarity, the law is *repressive*. Because people are very similar in this type of society, and because they tend to believe very strongly in the common morality, any offense against this value system is likely to be of significance to most individuals. Because most people believe deeply in the common morality, an offender is likely to be severely punished for any action that is considered an offense against the collective moral system (Durkheim, 1997).

In contrast, in societies with organic solidarity, the law is *restitutive*. Instead of being severely punished for even seemingly minor offenses against the collective morality, individuals in this more modern type of society are likely simply to be asked to comply with the law or to make restitution to those who have been harmed by their actions. Although some repressive laws exist in a society with organic solidarity, such as capital punishment, restitutive law is more characteristic of that group. There is no powerful and coercive common morality: a vast majority of people do not react emotionally to a breach of the law.

The monitoring of repressive law is in the hands of the masses in a society with mechanical solidarity, but the maintenance of the restitutive law is primarily the responsibility of specialized agencies, such as the courts or the police. Such a model is consistent with the increased division of labor in a society with organic solidarity (Durkheim, 1997).

Trust, Social Cohesion, and Social Relationships

The notion of trust is critical to the sociological understanding and conceptualization of society. It is also important in understanding the ability of people to develop some level of morality that guides their thinking, actions, and fulfilling their obligations and duties to each other. Only when such trust exists can a reasonable and meaningful social order emerge.

While the notion of trust in social relationships and its impact on society was initially outlined in Durkheim's work, Seligman (1998), who dedicates a significant portion of his book to analyzing Durkheim's ideas, suggests something different. Instead of arguing for increasing levels of trust among citizens, the modern society, with its significant and increasing role differentiation, results in a loss of trust. Seligman argues that the moral fabric of society that is created by the division of labor results in a less compelling collective conscience, where people base their trust on familiarity and function, not on any strong sense of morality or collective unity. Because people are not necessarily in agreement with a particular way of life, they increasingly rely on legal norms to promote societal problems as well as solving interactional conflicts. In other words, the strength of informal social control weakens as society evolves and there is greater reliance on formal mechanisms of control to guide people's behavior. A heavy reliance on formal social control also changes the general tone of social interaction, in that people may become more compliant with the rules, but they also generally become more focused on the letter of the law rather than on the larger intent of its creation.

In his book, *The Problem of Trust*, Seligman (1998) offers an illustration of this important point. As he describes, prior to the legal ban on smoking in public places, a man, a cigarette smoker, might typically ask patrons of a given area for permission to smoke there. In those instances where people did not want to be exposed to smoke, the man would likely refrain from doing so out of consideration for them as an attempt to coexist peacefully with others. However, once a ban on public smoking occurred, the man likely complied with the law and refrained from smoking in those areas where it was prohibited. However, in those areas where smoking was not restricted, the man would not likely feel the need to seek permission or honor the request of fellow patrons (because the law outlined the boundaries of where smoking was and was not permitted). Seligman argues that the rules and regulations regarding smoking established the notion of trust among citizens (because it was illegal to do so in certain spaces), but it was not based on any agreed upon social contract or consensus about what was appropriate or morally correct. What it also accomplished was to create a sense of legalism and a narrow definition of what constitutes trust.

Thus, much of the decline of trust in society is based on the idea that people dedicate an enormous amount of time attempting to find loopholes in the law rather than adhering to a sense of morality and trust in social relations. Seligman also argues that this reliance on legal norms to solve social disputes and problems has transformed the nature of trust away from agreed upon ideas to one that either focuses entirely too much on the letter of the law to define social interaction, or creates a climate of "gaming" the system, where people look for opportunities to skirt their obligations to others (Seligman, 1998).

Karen Cook's (2000) work, entitled *Trust in Society*, also offers important insight into the nature of trust. As part of a series on trust by the Russell Sage Foundation, in this edited collection of articles from sociologists, psychologists, political scientists, and economists, Cook's work explores the importance of trust in sustaining relationships and the process by which people decide to trust others. This is important as society increasingly becomes interdependent as a result of globalization, the need to trust others in a host of situations becomes imperative for everyone. More specifically, Cook's work explores the public's decreasing trust in physicians, attorneys, spiritual leaders, politicians, scientists, and teachers, which could have a significant impact on social life in the future. Thus, the breakdown of trust as a social phenomenon, along with the ways in which trust can be restored, is crucial to the sense of social cohesion of any society, but particularly in the United States.

Similarly, Hardin's (2002) book, *Trust and Trustworthiness*, examines how trust is engendered and the factors that lead people to trust others, including people's trust of institutions in society. Hardin's main argument is that we trust people based on our belief that they have strong reasons to act in our best interests. He refers to this trust as *encapsulated interest*. The logic, of course, is that the incentive for people to do this is due to the fact that they want an ongoing relationship with us. But social relationships can only be sustained when there is trust, meaning a reliance on others to do what they have promised in a given situation.

Most important, however, is the development of trustworthiness, which goes beyond a given transaction and moves toward the development of an ongoing relationship where parties can rely on others in a host of circumstances, especially when one party can be relied upon even if they do not benefit from a given transaction. It is only then that at a societal level can there be any meaningful sense of social solidarity and predictability in relationships.

TRUST AND THE CHIROPRACTIC PROFESSION

Durkheim's ideas about the collective conscience, social solidarity, and trust, along with insight offered by Cook, Hardin, and Seligman can be used in understanding the current state of affairs in the chiropractic profession. As has been noted throughout this study, there is a consistent theme of mistrust in the interaction with chiropractors, where about half of the population in the United States do not trust them. Even among those who regularly use chiropractors, there is some element of mistrust. As Connie, a chiropractic patient, stated,

> I have these mixed feelings about my chiropractor. I want to think that he is honest and acts ethically in treating patients, but I'd be lying if I said I didn't wonder at times if he was really being totally honest all of the time. I know a little about how insurance plans work, but I'm no expert. Still, it sometimes feels as though my chiropractor tries to push the boundaries a bit. Every time I come in, I get the same exact treatment no matter what I tell him is going on. And then he tells me that my insurance doesn't cover some of the treatments. It just makes me wonder if I really need that every single time.

The comments offered by this patient are reflective of those found among many other chiropractic patients interviewed in this study. While many stated they like their provider and believe he/she is helping them, at some level there is a concern about whether the chiropractor is really acting in their best interests. As Connie points out, some patients sometimes felt like they were being manipulated in some way, especially when it came to maintenance care.

The fact that many patients said they wondered if maintenance care was not a marketing strategy or an attempt to "churn" them raises questions about whether their chiropractor is completely trustworthy. It is not known, of course, but one wonders if these same patients would react similarly if their physician or dentist informed them of this development. Of course, as was noted, the data shows that people who do not see a chiropractor have trust issues with the profession, which may be the reason why they do not seek treatment from them. Again, this is not to say that chiropractors are not trustworthy, just that from the patient's point of view, there are questions about the extent and degree of that trust.

In addition to the provider–patient relationship, many chiropractors in the study noted they felt that physicians did not trust them. During the interviews, a common lament by chiropractors was that they felt discriminated against by doctors who will not refer patients to them for treatment. Other chiropractors believe that doctors understand the value and benefit of chiropractic medicine, but refuse to refer patients out of a fear that they would lose revenue from their own practices. Jim, a physician, sharply disagrees with this assessment. He says,

> Listen, while there was a lawsuit many years ago because the AMA tried to shut chiropractors down, there remains this feeling that all doctors are against chiropractors or that physicians somehow feel threatened by what they do. I don't feel threatened since they are not going to take away patients from me. . . . Some of the things that I do can't be done by chiropractors and even if they could, there's no way they are going to be a threat to me—I have more work than I know how to manage as it is. But this perception that the medical community is threatened by chiropractors and so we try to cut them out of the industry is all in their heads. Maybe that's what they do to each other or that's what they might do if they were in our position, but the problem really feels to me like an example of their own inferiority complexes and they are looking for someone to blame for the fact that they haven't done what they needed to in order for society and other professions to look at them with respect.
>
> This notion that we know what chiropractors do and the only reason we don't refer to them is because we don't want to lose the fee? That's nonsense. If we can find a way to help the patient, why wouldn't we explore that? I refer patients to physical therapists all the time, technically I'm "losing" money on that unless I own that PT practice. So it's not a matter of some conspiracy or we are so economically motivated that we want to cut people out of the business. We just don't know what business they are actually in and aren't able to get good answers when we ask them.

Many physicians who make referrals to chiropractors also raise some concerns. Questions about the wide variance in treatments and whether or not their patients would be exploited by unscrupulous providers create tension between the two groups. Many physicians, particularly specialists, do not feel they have the time or the inclination to discover whether a particular chiropractor takes a reasonable and effective approach to treating neck and back injuries, so they do not refer any patients for chiropractic care. As they say, this is not out of a fear of losing patients or a concerted effort to discriminate against them; rather it is due to the fact that the industry is not sufficiently regulated—there is a lack of trust of the profession or those in it.

Finally, there is mistrust within the profession. As was noted in the accounts by chiropractors themselves, chiropractors cannot seem to agree with each other at a collective level about issues relating to scope of practice, philosophy of treatment, or even whether the vertebral subluxation exists.

Providers have also talked about the dubious and outright fraudulent practices of their colleagues or the use of practice-building seminars that teach chiropractors how to make money, but not necessarily place patient care at the top of the priority list. Other providers talk about not sharing information with their colleagues out of a fear of them stealing their marketing tips and ideas, or of poaching patients and employees, who often take patients with them.

Still other chiropractors show a significant level of disdain and mistrust based on the issue of scope of practice or the splintering state of the profession, with some groups attempting to become more like primary care physicians, while others refuse to consider the importance of the evidence and research surrounding the existence of the vertebral subluxation.

The scope of mistrust within the profession is perhaps one of the most salient features of the study and while every provider or individual who participated in this project lamented the problem and the need to remedy it, chiropractors as a group do not seem willing to hold their colleagues accountable for misdeeds and continue to remain dislocated in their ability to reach any type of consensus in how to regulate the profession. The end result is that not only does the profession lack a meaningful identity, the public's understanding, along with the medical community's position, suggests that perhaps something is amiss with the entire industry.

It seems apparent from the accounts offered in this study that the need for autonomy is a critical component to understanding why so many providers are unwilling to allow their profession to be regulated. It also seems apparent that, in Durkheimian terms, there is no collective conscience and no real sense of solidarity and there remain questions about the trustworthiness of chiropractors by patients, the public, the medical community, and even among chiropractors themselves.

CONCLUSIONS AND SUMMARY OF FINDINGS

As was mentioned in the opening chapter, very little sociological research has been done on chiropractors or chiropractic medicine in the last two decades. The present study attempts to address this issue and there were several notable themes that emerged as the project unfolded. While there remain significant challenges in medicine that will likely continue in the foreseeable future, there were a number of unique issues that were discovered in the study of chiropractors. Even though these were mentioned in previous chapters, because of their significance, particularly as they relate to the future of the profession, they are worth mentioning again here.

Perceptions of Chiropractors

Several times during the study, chiropractors made reference to the fact that physicians do not like them, discriminate against them for various reasons, or feel as though they are misunderstood by doctors. In response, every physician or specialist interviewed in this study pointed out that the problem was not that physicians did not like chiropractors, but rather they could not trust them to treat a patient based on sound principles.

Physicians also scoffed at the idea that they refrained from referring patients to chiropractors out of fear of losing revenue or patients—most indicated that they had too many patients to begin with and would not feel the effects of "losing" them by making a referral to a chiropractor. Instead, the concern was that they could not reliably know what a chiropractor might do to a patient because there is no consistency in the care provided by chiropractors, nor have there been efforts by the profession to self-regulate its unethical colleagues—and they did not want their patients exploited or injured as a result.

Chiropractors in this study also point to some level of persecution by insurance companies—indicating that others in medicine engage in inappropriate billing and fraud, but that insurance companies target chiropractors because of their limited ability to stand up to them. While there may be some truth to these criticisms, there is also evidence to indicate that the identification of chiropractors for audits may be justified. As was mentioned in the last chapter, a recent report by the Office of Inspector General, a division of the U.S. Department of Health and Human Services, the agency responsible for overseeing health programs like Medicare and Medicaid, of all the providers who were cited for fraud, abuse, and errors in Medicare billing, chiropractors were overwhelmingly the largest set of offenders.

From the accounts by Medicare authorities, and from chiropractors as well, the crux of the issue appears to be the limits insurance companies like

Medicare are placing on chiropractic treatments, including the number of visits allowed per year and the use of maintenance care. This remains controversial, as chiropractors argue that the insurance companies do not know what is the best course of treatment for their patients, while insurance companies contend that providers are misusing the system and ignoring federal guidelines. As one chiropractor in this study pointed out, many chiropractors continue to bill, sometimes fraudulently, either in the hopes of not getting caught or perhaps with a misguided belief that they can persuade insurance companies that what they are doing is not maintenance care.

Identity Issues in Chiropractic Medicine

The topic of a professional identity in chiropractic medicine largely speaks to the internal strife and an inability or unwillingness to find common ground that would provide some level of legitimacy and credibility to chiropractors. The distinctive types identified in the literature, Straights, Mixers, and Reformers, call attention to this fragmentation, but the problem may be even more rudimentary: the vertebral subluxation. The debate continues, with some groups making an effort to document the existence and successful treatment of subluxations, while others claim it to be a historical development better left to the archives since it has not been, and likely cannot be, proven to exist.

Still, almost every chiropractor in this study tells a story of remarkable healing. The explanation for these events can be related to the powerful impact of suggestion, the placebo effect, or something else. While it is true that miracles occur in medicine, such events do not necessarily validate the treatments provided. In fact, some might argue that the miracle occurred *in spite* of the treatments given to patients. Claims by chiropractors that their treatment of a subluxation cured a disease can be seen as similar to faith healers, who are convinced that their prayers caused the person to be healed (see, for instance, Hanegraaff, 2012). In the same way that faith healers use these examples to "prove" the effectiveness of their work, it is far from a sure thing and may cause people to remain skeptical of them. Similarly, chiropractors who make outlandish claims about the effectiveness of chiropractic treatment, or who rely on faulty data, will likely be seen in a similar way.

The Costs of Health Care in the United States

While this may not be a new idea or suggestion, the changes in medicine, including the escalating costs, which translate into higher out-of-pocket expenses to the average patient, accelerate the need for the establishment of trust on a wider scale for all medical providers.

As was mentioned, in a 2016 report by the U.S. Department of Health and Human Services (DHHS), health care spending is growing at a faster rate than the national economy. Growth is expected to average about 5.8 percent from 2015 to 2025. National expenditures for health care were $3.35 trillion in 2016, which is approximately $10,345 for every man, woman, and child in the United States. These expenditures represented about 18 percent of the U.S. Gross Domestic Product in 2015. The rise in health care costs is expected to increase to 20 percent of the economy by 2025 (Alonzo-Zandivar, 2016).

The DHHS report also points to the specialization of medicine as a contributor to the escalating costs, along with the aging of America, where Medicare and Medicaid are expected to grow more rapidly than private insurance as the population ages. In fact, by 2025, the government will account for 47 percent of all health care spending. However, the larger numbers of people eligible for care does not tell the entire story. The DHHS estimates that about 5 percent of the population account for nearly half of the health care spending in a given year. This means that even with affordable health care for everyone, its use will remain significantly uneven (Alonzo-Zandivar, 2016).

The escalating costs in health care, along with the declining reimbursements by insurance companies, could have a potentially devastating effect on chiropractors. For those providers already struggling financially, the continuation along this pathway could result in many providers deciding to close their practices. As was discovered in the statistical analysis of the data from the licensure board in South Carolina, there is already some evidence to support this trend: there has been a 39 percent decrease in the number of chiropractors who renewed their licenses between 2016 and 2017.

One might argue that this finding is the result of a large group of chiropractors deciding to retire from the profession, but it may also be the result of providers experiencing financial difficulties. The interview data in this study supports both possible conclusions, but a common theme in this study were the laments by chiropractors who complained about the inability to remain in practice due to health care reform and the intense competition for patients.

As patients' out-of-pocket expenses increase, it is imaginable that they may decide to engage in their own form of triage and use their resources to address the more immediate medical needs that cannot be addressed without the services of a physician or specialist. Such a strategy could potentially result in a significant loss of revenue for chiropractors, particularly if patients question the trustworthiness of their provider or of the treatments offered.

The "Practice" of Chiropractic Medicine

While many providers complained about the ability to sustain their practice, citing concerns about reimbursement issues and competition between colleagues, it is fair to say that chiropractors themselves need to accept some of the responsibility for their plight. Again, while not all chiropractors in this study struggled financially; some claim to be doing quite well and have a thriving practice. However, this was more the exception rather than the rule. Instead, most chiropractors in this study stated they struggled to make ends meet, with some even eliminating staff positions in an effort to reduce overhead. This means that the administrative work falls to the providers in addition to treating patients. This, coupled with the increasing demands required by insurance companies to document patient treatment plans, can easily create an environment in which the chiropractor carries a heavy workload both inside and outside the office. Given that many providers claim insufficient preparation or insight into successfully operating a practice, it is not surprising to witness many chiropractors struggling to stay afloat, with no real end in sight in terms of achieving success.

That said, there are some elements found in the analysis of chiropractic practices that do not require any advanced business acumen or expertise. In fact, what is perhaps most surprising is that so many chiropractors who complained of declining revenue and patient census remain committed to the idea of running their practice on a three-day-per-week schedule. It is hard to imagine any small business person not recognizing that if they are not attracting more customers they would not consider extending their hours of operation or changing them to meet customer needs. Every chiropractor interviewed in this study talked extensively about how much they cared about their patients and their concern about their well-being; however when it came to remaining open longer so patients can come to the office after working hours or opening on Saturdays, virtually all of the providers interviewed in this study either dismissed that as an ineffective strategy or claimed they tried it at one time or another with little success.

It is worthy of note, however, that most who attempted such a strategy did not actually employ it for more than a couple of months and only informed their existing patients of this change. As was noted earlier, the patients who regularly visited the office likely did so because normal hours were convenient for them. It is unreasonable to expect the scheduling changes to impact that segment of the population. And because other patients or potential customers were not notified (meaning it was not a part of the marketing strategy), how reasonable is it that any success would occur? This, of course, even assumes that any type of marketing strategy existed. Many providers noted that they had Facebook pages or that they ran ads in alternative publications occasionally, but that was essentially all the marketing that occurred.

Similarly, for those providers who were unwilling to modify their hours of operation, another challenge was that even when the office operated under a traditional model, it often included two- and a half-hour lunch breaks. This means that, routinely, chiropractic offices were closed from 12:30 pm to 3 pm. If a patient wanted to be seen on their lunch hour, the office was closed. Many primary care physicians and family medicine practices close for lunch for an hour, but it is usually from 1 to 2 pm, to allow those patients who needed to be seen to come in during their lunch break. Not so with chiropractors. In response, chiropractors claim they need this extended time for their physical recovery because treating patients places a heavy demand on their bodies. While that may be true, and also debatable depending on the type of treatments provided, other professions are physically taxing—roofing, landscaping, restaurant work, construction—but workers in those professions operate on a forty-hour week or more and lunch breaks may only be thirty minutes.

Most people who own a business recognize that the endeavor cannot be seen as a part-time job, with long lunches and no weekends or holidays. To do so means that customers will find another way to have their needs met. Perhaps chiropractors felt that they have a closed system, where all providers operate under such a model. However, the Joint is changing that—where they are open on weekends and after hours and only close on Christmas and other significant holidays.

Thus, it is difficult to consider the argument made by many chiropractors in this study, and perhaps those outside of it, who complain about not making enough money, when they simply are not putting in the time needed to grow a business. Perhaps this is a result of something that Kat pointed out in one of our conversations. She said that the way the profession was "sold" to her was that she was going to be able to work part-time and still make six figures, unlike physicians who would be required to take call and dedicate a lot of time to the practice of medicine. Somewhere in the development of the profession, it seems the culture adopted a complacency that is no longer relevant to today's consumers and if they want to remain a viable option in the treatment of patients, chiropractors are going to have to be more visible and available when patients need them.

The Future of Chiropractic Medicine

As was noted in the chapter on health care reform, it does not appear that medicine can remain on its current fee for service pathway. Given that much of the cost of medicine in this country is attributed to high fees by physicians and the specialization in the industry, insurance companies, as part of a managed care model, will ensure that reimbursements become smaller and smaller and more narrowly define the treatments. A potential consequence of this approach, of course, is that many chiropractors will simply stop taking insurance and go to a cash model, where the patient pays for the treatment.

This is the business model adopted by the Joint and it is possible that a much greater segment of medicine will adopt this approach in the future. However, the risk is that such an approach will result in only a small segment of the population using chiropractic treatments. A cash model will also exclude a relatively large segment of the population who cannot afford these payments. This can easily result in chiropractors raising their fees to capitalize on the small group who make use of their services and it will also likely increase the competition between providers, causing an assortment of challenges within the profession.

Informed consumers may also discover, as the research shows, that chiropractic treatments are not any better than conventional remedies and provide only a marginal benefit for some patients. Thus, faced with taking a mild pain killer, using ice and resting, patients might opt for that as a solution to routine back and neck pain. Thus, while there may be some who cling to the dogma and belief that chiropractic works, and there will be some for whom the extra expense is worth the immediate relief from pain and the lack of mobility, the future does not look bright for a profession that cannot seem to get out of its own way and define a segment of the health care marketplace.

Chiropractic medicine could end up like Jimmy, one chiropractor who said if chiropractic loses its place in medicine, he "wants to go down swinging," meaning clinging to the traditional idea of straight chiropractic. However, it does not have to be that way. Rather, the industry has to realize its contributions to medicine are made by others who are equally competent and can adequately perform. Many of chiropractic techniques being employed and validated under the rubric of "evidence-based" are actually developed by used in other professions, such as physical therapy, giving them greater credibility than chiropractic medicine.

This is especially true if the problems people experience cannot be linked to vertebrae but rather to muscular issues that limit joint mobility. As one chiropractor pointed out, emphatically stating that massage therapy is not chiropractic medicine, even though some of those treatments can result in the same outcome: the muscles to relax and the joint regains some mobility. In the end, chiropractic treatment may end up being a technical form of treatment that is a bit different from physical therapy (which will continue to focus on stretching and strengthening exercises), while chiropractors may become pain management technicians who eschew drugs as a primary form of treatment.

Even chiropractors offer the observation that if people take better care of themselves and strengthen the muscles around the back, many of thechallenges they face will be greatly minimized. This is not to say that a regular exercise program and better nutrition will solve every problem, but there is ample research that shows it goes a long way in preventing many health-related problems. Of course, people who are active are likely to sustain injuries from time to time, but one does not have to be an aggressive athlete to maintain good health. Unfortunately, many Americans do not seem to want to take reasonable and necessary steps to remain healthy. Instead, they generally eat poorly, fail to exercise, and then need some type of intervention when they experience pain. Modern medicine has responded to these demands of complacency by developing medications to alleviate symptoms and pain, but what is likely needed in most cases is a reasonably disciplined approach to an active lifestyle. Unfortunately, as long as people can take a pill and solve their problems, they will likely take the path of least resistance and effort.

In the end, chiropractic treatments can be shaped to fit into the larger wellness paradigm and that may be why some people find it an attractive alternative to other forms of treatment. However, using chiropractic care to occasionally alleviate pain is not the same as suggesting that chiropractic treatment fixes all health-related problems or cures diseases like cancer, asthma, colic in babies, or other significant issues, nor is chiropractic care the only way to address general symptoms relating to pain. That is, the evidence shows that there are other equally effective modalities that yield the same results that are far less expensive (Qaseem et al., 2017).

One way to consider the value of chiropractic treatment is to view it like all forms of medical treatment: it is one option among several to consider in addressing the problem of pain management. For those patients who are not eligible for other types of treatment or who would not likely maintain or follow a course of treatment, such as physical therapy, stretching exercises, or an exercise program that requires a dedication and commitment to its success, chiropractic may offer relief of pain and symptoms.

Sociologically, the study of chiropractic medicine and chiropractors offers us great insight into the nature of social relationships and interaction, and linkages to important social issues such as health care, trust and social cohesion within the medical profession.

REFERENCES

Alonzo-Zaldivar, R. (2016). "$10,345 per person: U.S. health care spending reaches new peak." *Associated Press*, July 13th, available at http://www.pbs.com/newshour/rundown/new-peak-us-heaht-care-spending-10345-per-person/

Cook, K. 2001. *Trust in Society*. New York: Russell Sage Foundation.

Durkheim, E. 1997. *The Division of Labor in Society*. New York: Simon and Schuster.

———. 1897. *Suicide*. New York: The Free Press.

Festinger, L. 1954. "A Theory of Social Comparison Processes." *Journal of Human Relations* 7(2): 117–140.

Hanegraaff, H. 2012. *Christianity in Crisis: 21st Century*. Chicago, IL: Thomas Nelson.

Hardin H. 2002. *Trust and Trustworthiness*. New York: Russell Sage Foundation.

Heider, F. 1958. *The Psychology of Interpersonal Relations*. Hillsdale, NJ: Laurence Erlbaum Associates.

Qaseem, A., Wilt, T. J., McClean, R. M., and Forciea, M. A. (2017). "Non-Invasive Treatment for Acute, Subacute, and Chronic Low Back Pain: A Clinical Practice Guideline from the American College of Physicians." *Annals of Internal Medicine* 166: 514–530.

ReportLinker, 2017. *Alternative Medicine Industry in the U.S.—Forecast 2017.* Available at https://www.reportlinker.com/ci02242/Alternative-Medicine.html

Seligman, A. B. 1997. *The Problem of Trust*. Princeton, NJ: Princeton University Press.

Index

About the Author

Robert Hartmann McNamara is professor of criminal justice at The Citadel. He is the author of nearly thirty books including *Multiculturalism, Crime and Criminal Justice; Juvenile Delinquency: Linking Theory to Practice; Sociology as Every Day Life*; *Homelessness in America*, 3 vols.; *The Lost Population: Status Offenders in America*; *Boundary Dwellers: Homeless Women in Transitional Housing; A New Look at American Society; Perspectives on Social Problems; Understanding Contemporary Social Problems; Crossing the Line: Interracial Couples in the South*; *Crime Displacement: The Other Side of Prevention*; *The Times Square Hustler: Male Prostitution in New York City*; *Sex, Scams and Street Life: The Sociology of New York City's Times Square; Beating the Odds: Crime, Poverty, and Life in the Inner City; Police and Policing*; *The Urban Landscape: Selected Readings*; and *Social Gerontology*. Dr. McNamara is the former associate provost and dean of the Graduate College at The Citadel, as well as the founding associate dean of its Evening Undergraduate Studies program. He is also the founding director of the 2 plus 2 program in criminal justice. Dr. McNamara also served as a senior research fellow for the National Strategy Information Center, the Police Executive Research Forum, and the Pacific Institute for Research and Evaluation. He has extensive leadership experience and served as an American Council of Education's Emerging Leaders Fellow in 2015 and completed the Association of Private Colleges and Universities Leadership Program in 2016.

Dr. McNamara has also been a consultant for state, federal, and private agencies on topics such as AIDS, drug abuse, urban redevelopment, homelessness, policing, gangs, and health care. He worked with the Regional Community Policing Institute at Eastern Kentucky University to study school safety in eight high schools across the state. He also worked with the Mexican government and the National Strategy Information Center to develop an anti-corruption curriculum in their public schools. Dr. McNamara holds a PhD in sociology from Yale University.

www.ingramcontent.com/pod-product-compliance
Ingram Content Group UK Ltd.
Pitfield, Milton Keynes, MK11 3LW, UK
UKHW041125071026
15587UKWH00009B/239

9 781498 591409